ATLAS *of* TOTAL HIP 'REPLACEMENT

ORTHOPAEDIC SURGICAL SKILLS

Series Editor

ANDREW J. WEILAND, M.D
Professor
Department of Orthopaedic Surgery
Cornell University Medical College
Attending Orthopaedic Surgeon
Department of Hand and Orthpaedic Surgery
The Hospital for Special Surgery
New York, New York

Forthcoming

Operative Shoulder Surgery
Stephen Copeland, F.R.C.S.

Atlas of Knee Surgery
Russell L. Windsor, M.D.

ATLAS *of* TOTAL HIP REPLACEMENT

PAUL M. PELLICCI, M.D.

Associate Attending Orthopaedic Surgeon
Co-Director
The Hip Clinic
The Hospital for Special Surgery
Associate Professor of Surgery
Assistant Professor of Cell Biology and Anatomy
Cornell University Medical College
New York, New York

DOUGLAS E. PADGETT, M.D.

Assistant Professor of Surgery
Cornell University Medical College
Assistant Attending Surgeon
Department of Orthopaedic Surgery
Attending Surgeon
The Hip Clinic
The Hospital for Special Surgery
New York, New York

Illustrations by
VIRGINIA FERRANTE, M.A.

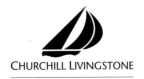

CHURCHILL LIVINGSTONE

New York, Edinburgh, London, Melbourne, San Francisco, Tokyo

Library of Congress Cataloging-in-Publication Data

Pellicci, Paul.
    Atlas of total hip replacement / Paul M. Pellicci, Douglas E.
  Padgett ; illustrations by Virginia Ferrante.
       p. cm — (Orthopaedic surgical skills)
    Includes index.
    ISBN 0-443-08902-7
    1. Total hip replacement—Atlases.   I. Padgett, Douglas E.
  II. Title.   III. Series.
   [DNLM: 1. Hip Prosthesis—atlases. 2. Hip Joint—surgery
 —atlases. WE 17 P391a 1995]
  RD549.P44 1995
  617.5′810592—dc20
  DNLM/DLC
  for Library of Congress

95-9614

CIP

Distributed in the United Kingdom by Churchill Livingstone, Robert Stevenson House, 1–3 Baxter's Place, Leith Walk, Edinburgh EH1 3AF, and by associated companies, branches, and representatives throughout the world.

Accurate indications, adverse reactions, and dosage schedules for drugs are provided in this book, but it is possible that they may change. The reader is urged to review the package information data of the manufacturers of the medications mentioned.

The Publishers have made every effort to trace the copyright holders for borrowed material. If they have inadvertently overlooked any, they will be pleased to make the necessary arrangements at the first opportunity.

Acquisitions Editor: *Jennifer Mitchell*
Production Editor: *Kamely Dahir*
Production Supervisor: *Laura Mosberg Cohen*
Desktop Coordinator: *Jo-Ann Demas*
Cover Design: *Jeannette Jacobs*

Printed in the United States of America

First published in 1995   7 6 5 4 3 2 1

Foreword

The Orthopaedic Surgical Skills series was conceived as a vehicle through which experts in the various subspecialties in orthopaedic surgery could present common surgical procedures to a broad orthopaedic audience. The authors of this series are well regarded, both nationally and internationally, in their specific fields. Each author will thoroughly present a surgical technique used commonly by orthopaedic surgeons. These atlases are, in essence, step-by-step operative notes.

One of the merits of starting a surgical atlas series is to recognize the changing nature of surgery and to relate in a clear and concise manner many of the newest advances within the field. In addition, the advent of the series will note the consequences, changes, and impact of recent technical developments. We feel that the *Atlas* is an ideal platform with which to illustrate and acknowledge such changes by combining succinct text with clear illustrations.

Churchill Livingstone is committed to a strong art program and, for each atlas, has contracted one artist to observe the various surgical procedures in the operating room. By using a consistent, one artist source, we have insured the quality of the illustrations and helped to emphasize and highlight the authors' technique.

It is the goal of the series to further the education of surgeons and to improve their surgical techniques and end results.

Andrew J. Weiland, M.D.

Preface

The medical arena surrounding hip arthroplasty continues to change dramatically. Orthopaedic surgeons need to be aware of these fluctuations within their field and to be able to recognize and adopt important innovations while retaining established methods.

The role of cement fixation of the acetabular component has diminished considerably over the past decade. To put this in perspective, less than one percent of the acetabular components we have inserted since 1986 have been cemented. However, there are relative indications for cement fixation which include extreme advanced age, significant bone disease, and the inability to achieve initial stability of a cementless socket.

Accordingly, we urge our contemporaries to continue to acknowledge that success of the surgical procedure is attributable to correct preoperative examination and diagnosis. Failure can result when treatment is applied inappropriately. Meticulous preoperative analysis is essential to responsible patient care.

The Atlas of Total Hip Replacement presents a thorough and exact approach to both cemented and cementless fixation. Both procedures are detailed from opening to wound closure and are accompanied by clear and specific figures. While presenting a step-by-step guide to the procedures, we hope to provide fellow surgeons with instructions and information they will find relevant to the circumstances of their practice.

Paul M. Pellicci, M.D.
Douglas E. Padgett, M.D.

Contents

1

Preparation and Draping

X-ray with Overlying Template

The goal of total hip arthroplasty is to restore the normal hip biomechanics, provide adequate hip stability, and correct any leg length inequality. Clinical assessment of leg length inequality is essential prior to performing total hip arthroplasty. The discrepancy should be confirmed with preoperative radiographic measurements. The use of acetate overlay templates is helpful in achieving the goals of a successful total hip arthroplasty. The technique of templating should begin with the acetabular component. The ideal acetabular component is placed at the level of the radiographic teardrop with the component abducted approximately 40 degrees. This should allow for adequate containment of the acetabular component by host bone. At this point, the center of rotation of the acetabular component should be marked on the radiograph.

Femoral component templating must take into account variables such as proximal femoral deformity, femoral offset, and the ability to obtain adequate component fill of the femur. When employing a cemented femoral component, an adequate cement mantle of 2 to 3 mm should be obtained to maximize component fixation. Radiographic measurement of the lesser trochanter to center of rotation distance on the uninvolved hip is a useful guide to determining the distance to be reproduced at the time of surgery on the involved side. This lesser trochanter to center of rotation distance as well as restoration of femoral offset will determine the level of femoral neck resection. Finally, noticing the relationship of the tip of the greater trochanter to the center of rotation of the unaffected hip and whether this point is at, above, or below the center of rotation is a useful landmark to confirm at the time of reconstruction.

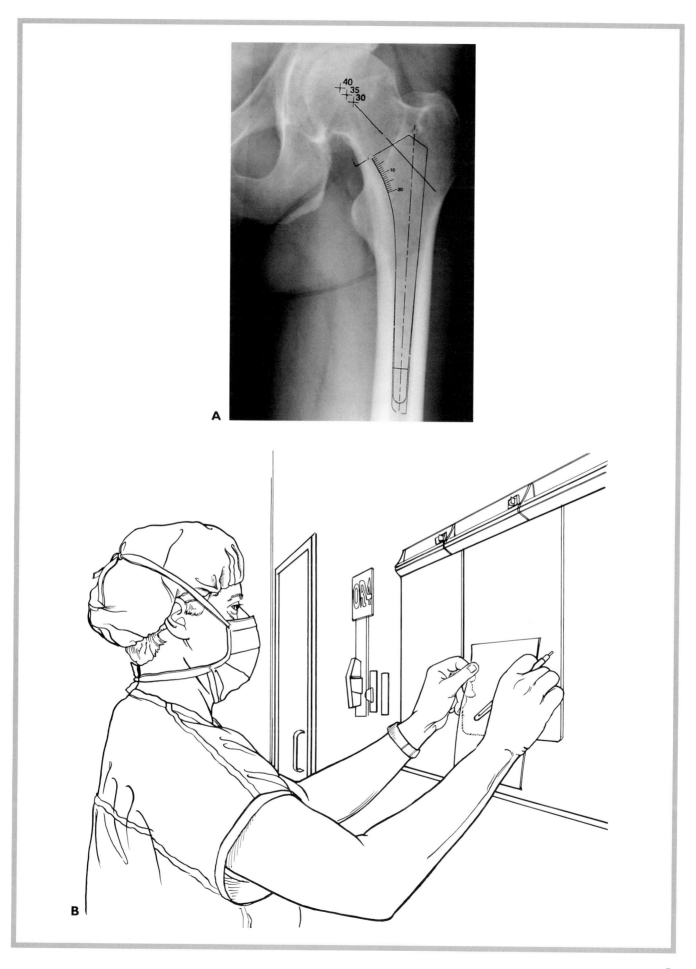

A

B

Total Body Exhaust Suits

The surgeon and surgical team wear total body exhaust suits to mini-mize the risk of infection. It is recommended that each member of the team wear two sets of gloves. The outer set of gloves should be changed after draping and a new outer set of gloves applied.

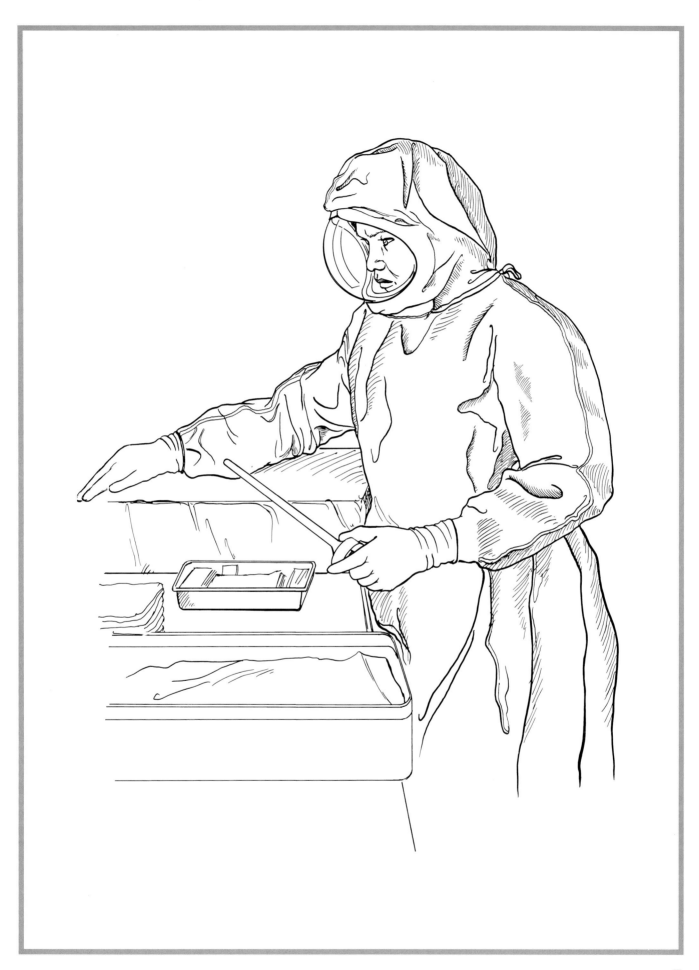

Anesthesia Position and Monitoring

A.

For the posterolateral approach, the patient is placed in the lateral decubitus position. Epidural anesthesia is the preferred method of anesthesia employed due to its hypotensive effects and overall lower rates of morbidity and mortality. Intraoperative monitoring with the use of arterial and central venous lines is routinely employed. The use of a first generation cepholosporin preoperatively and for 24 hours postoperatively is recommended as an antibiotic prophylaxis to reduce the risk of sepsis.

B.

A pulse oximeter, placed on the toe of the downside limb, monitors pulse and oxygenation. Excess pressure from the anterior and posterior pelvic pads can compromise blood flow to the down limb.

C.

Anterior and posterior pelvic pads stabilize the patient. A scapular pad augments stability. A supplemental pad of a softer type material, such as a "jelly-roll" placed in the subaxillary region, minimizes pressure on the chest wall and avoids injury to the neurovascular structures of the brachial plexus.

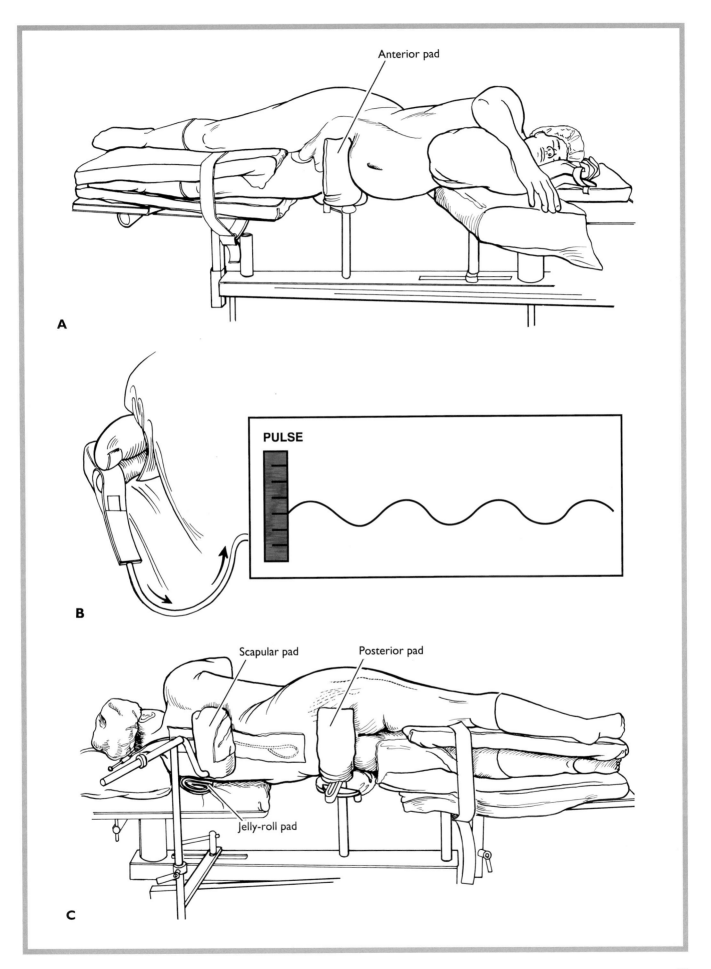

Anterior pad

A

PULSE

B

Scapular pad   Posterior pad

Jelly-roll pad

C

7

Area Draping and Environment

The operative environment is completely enclosed by plexiglass shields and plastic drapes that isolate the operative field from the anesthesia team. The use of laminar flow minimizes the traffic into and out of the operating room. A small window is kept open at the far end of the operative field to allow access to instruments and supplies.

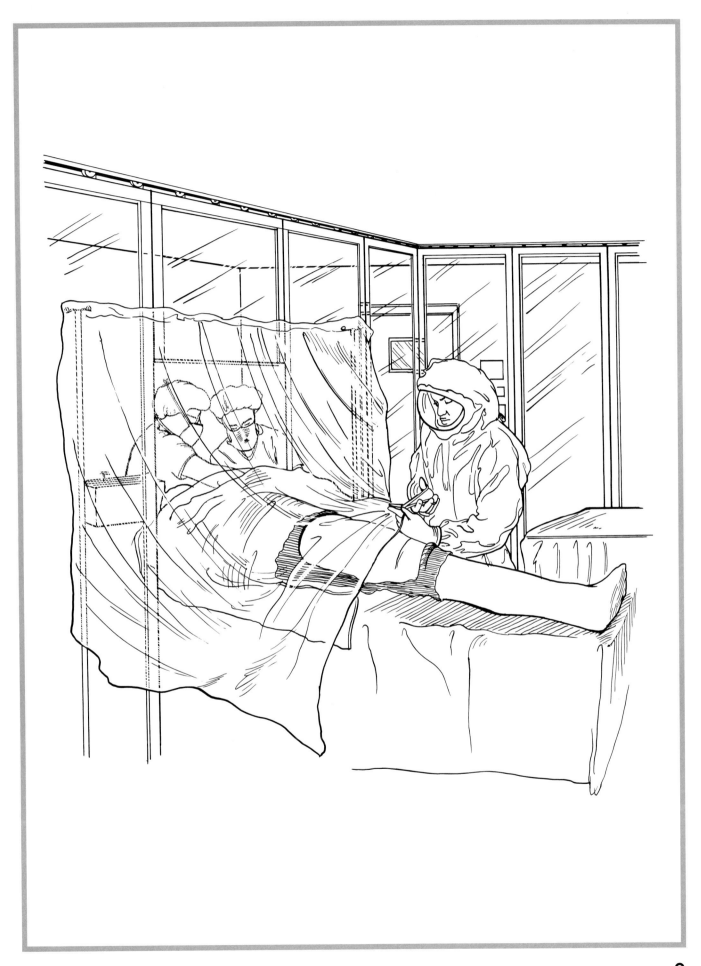

Draping

The operative leg remains free. The skin is thoroughly swabbed with an iodine based solution. Split sheets are placed below the patient. The leg is wrapped with second sheet and then placed in the stockinette still held extended in the air. After all sheets are placed, the operative site is wiped clean and dried. At this time, the skin may be marked for incision. The exposed skin is then covered with an iodine impregnated adhesive plastic sheet to seal the surrounding area.

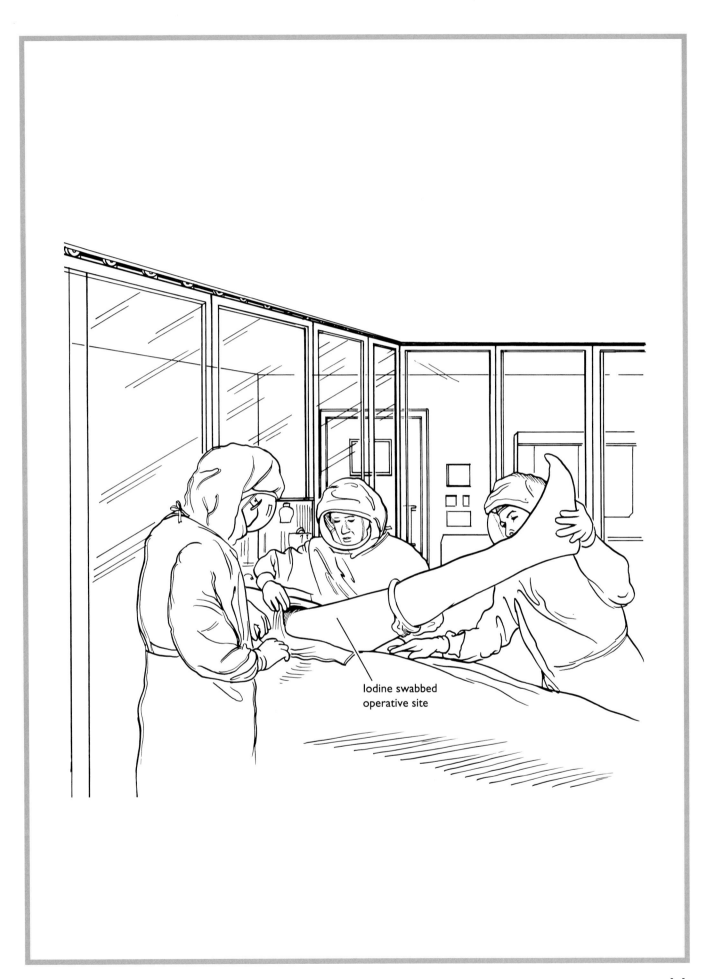

Iodine swabbed
operative site

2

Posterolateral Approach

Incision

The surgeon marks the skin at the posterior area of the greater trochanter and the posterior side of the shaft at the insertion point of the gluteus maximus tendon. The two points are connected by a straight line. The initial incision is made across the posterior corner of the greater trochanter from the center of the femoral shaft and is directed toward the sciatic notch. This incision is continued down through the skin and the subcutaneous layer down to the level of the fascia overlying the gluteus maximus and fascia lata. Electrocautery is used to coagulate bleeding blood vessels.

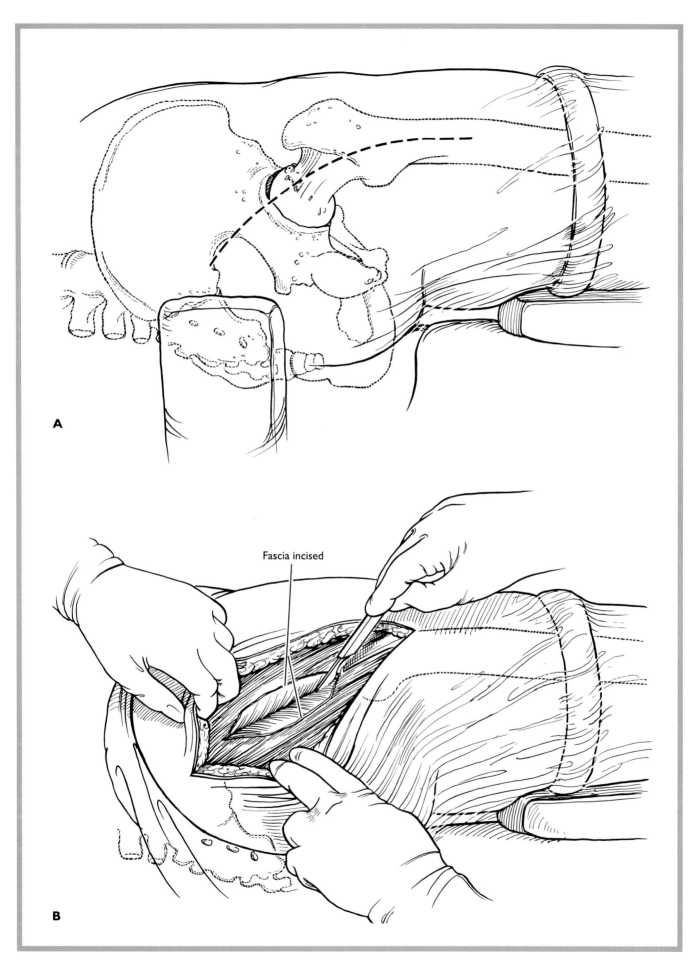

A

Fascia incised

B

15

Superficial Dissection

At this point, the fascia of the gluteus maximus and the fascia lata are incised. The fibers of the gluteus maximus are split bluntly in a superior and slightly posterior direction. Electrocautery is used to secure hemostasis.

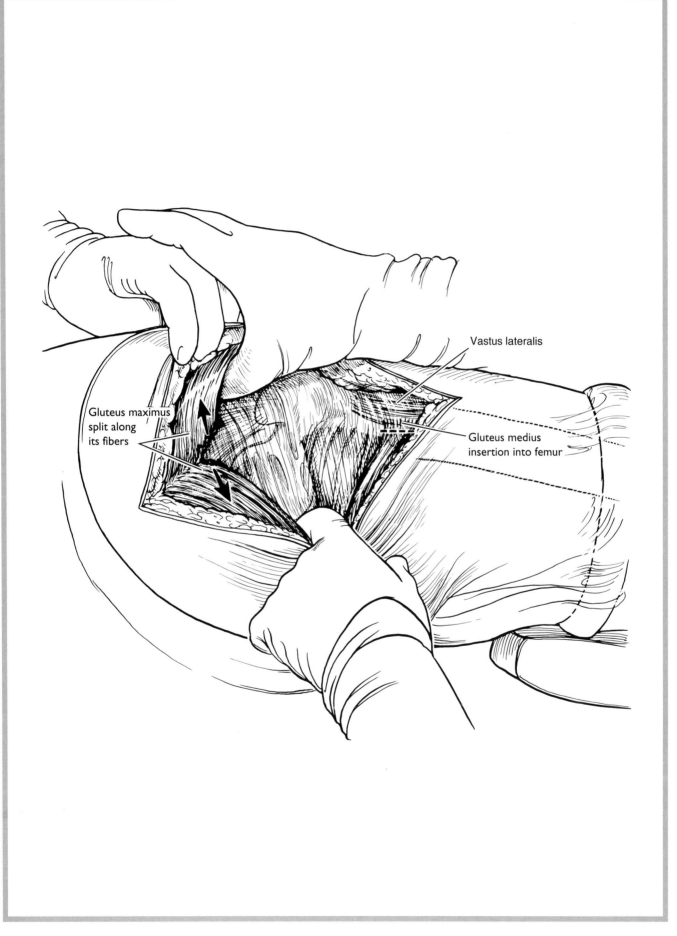

Vastus lateralis

Gluteus maximus
split along
its fibers

Gluteus medius
insertion into femur

17

Gluteus Maximus Insertion and Bursa

Antibiotic-soaked lap sponges are now sutured to the fascial edges. A self-retaining retractor (Charnley) can be inserted to facilitate exposure. The femoral insertion of the gluteus maximus tendon is now released using the electrocautery. Care is taken to identify all perforating branches of the profunda femoris artery that are often just beneath this tendinous insertion. The proximal 80 percent of the tendon is released. Holding the leg in slight internal rotation allows the sciatic nerve to fall posteriorly during this portion of the procedure and prevents injury to it. The greater trochanteric bursa is incised from the posterior fibers of the gluteus medius (landmark for the superior femoral neck) to the superior fibers of the quadratus femoris (defining the inferior extent of the femoral neck).

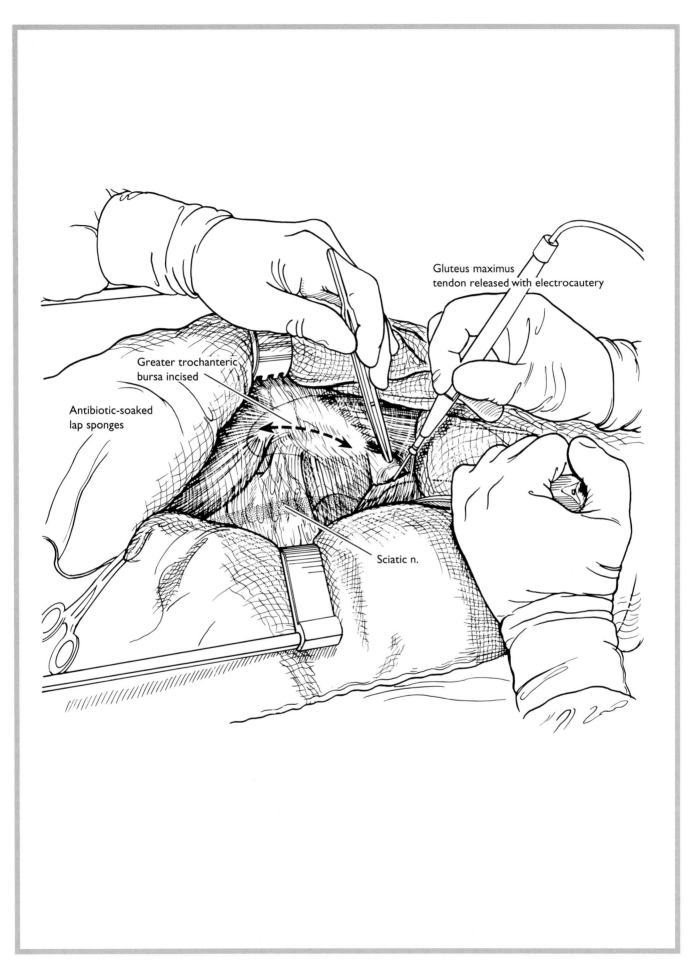

Gluteus maximus
tendon released with electrocautery

Greater trochanteric
bursa incised

Antibiotic-soaked
lap sponges

Sciatic n.

19

Retractors

A.

The piriformis tendon is identified just beneath the gluteus minimis tendon. An angled retractor (Hohmann) is placed superficial to the piriformis and deep to the gluteus minimis tendon above the superior neck of the femur to expose the superior capsule.

B.

A wider blunt tipped retractor (Aufranc) is placed just proximal to the quadratus femoris fibers to expose the inferior capsule.

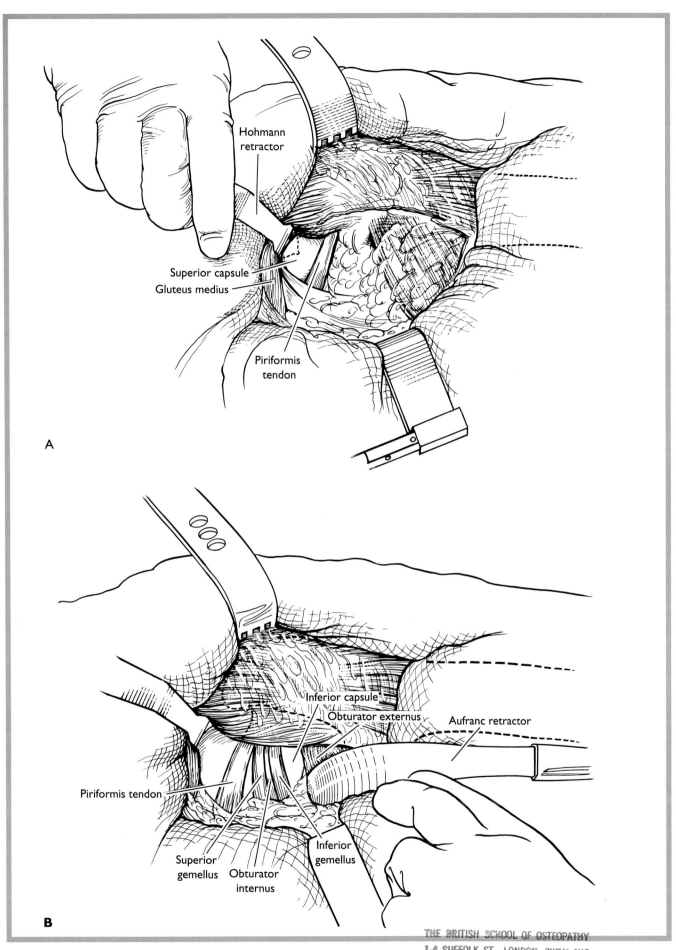

A

B

External Rotators and Capsulotomy

A.

The fibrofatty tissue overlying the external rotators is gently brushed posteriorly. The numerous venous anastomoses are electrocoagulated. With the femur extended and internally rotated the sciatic nerve will lie posteriorly, but its proximity must be kept in mind. The piriformis tendon and conjoined tendon (gemelli and obturator internus) are detached at their insertion using the electrocautery. They are tagged with nonabsorbable 1 sutures for later reattachment.

B.

The obturator externus tendon (lying inferiorly and deep to the quadratus) is released with the electrocautery. These structures are not tagged for later reattachment. An ascending branch of the medial femoral circumflex vein under cover of the quadratus should be identified and electrocoagulated.

C.

The posterior capsule is incised from the tip of the Hohmann retractor to the tip of the Aufranc retractor. A posterior "T" incision is made cutting from the acetabular rim anteriorly to meet the longitudinal incision. The release of soft tissue before dislocation helps to protect against femur fracture.

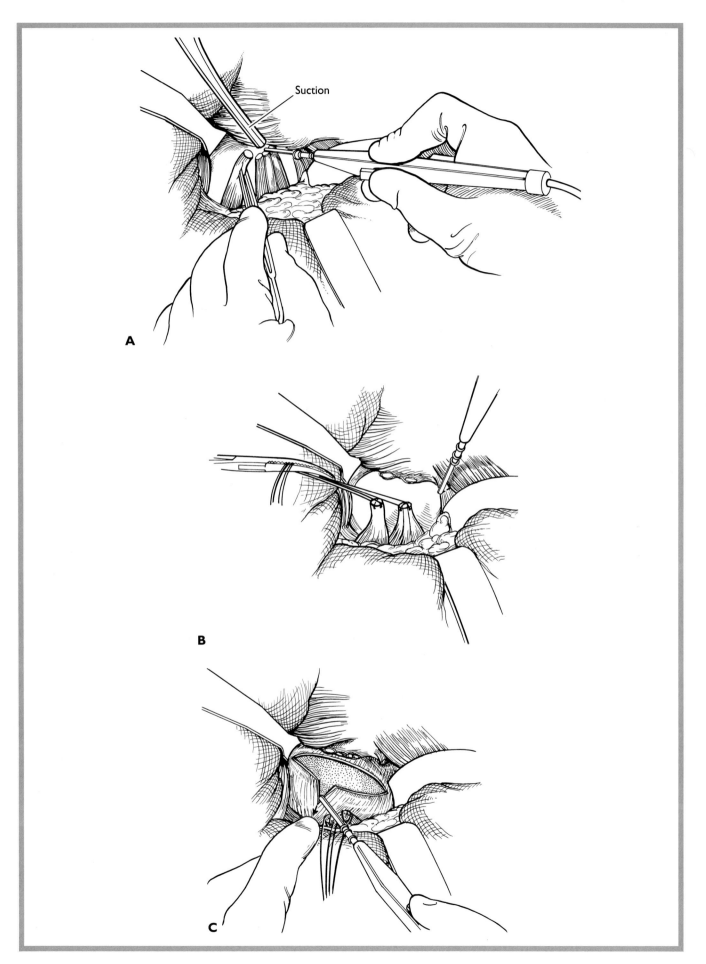

Suction

A

B

C

23

3

Femoral Dislocation and Osteotomy

Dislocation

A.

The hip is dislocated posteriorly by flexing the femur to a 90-degree angle, then adducting and internally rotating it as far as necessary.

B.

In a very stiff hip, more capsule superiorly may need to be resected. Additionally, the proximal fibers of the quadratus can be released from the posterior neck at this time using electrocautery. If large posterior osteophytes block dislocation, they should be placed osteomized. If dislocation is still difficult, a neck hook should be placed around the femoral neck and the head "pulled" out of the acetabulum. This technique should always be considered in a patient with thin femoral cortices where the torque involved with the dislocation maneuver can fracture the femur.

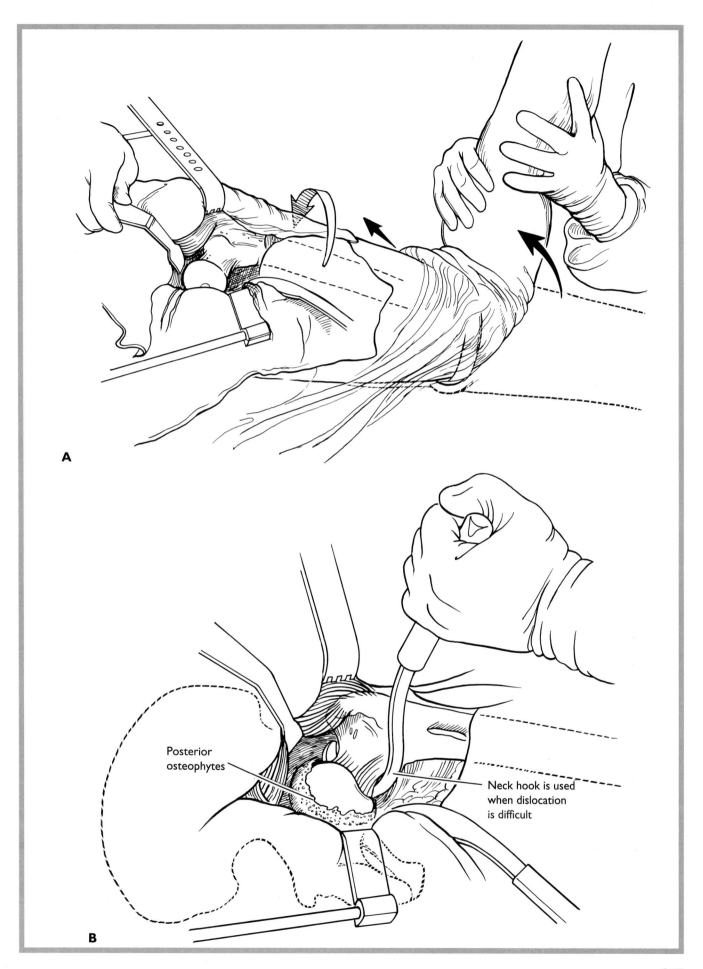

A

Posterior
osteophytes

Neck hook is used
when dislocation
is difficult

B

27

Exposure of the Posterior Femoral Neck

A.

After dislocation, the thigh is fully extended. The posterior aspect of the femoral neck is skeletonized to the lesser trochanter. In some instances, it may be necessary to release 2 to 3 mm of iliopsoas insertion to allow for accurate measurements from the lesser trochanter.

B.

The superior femoral neck is then protected by an angled retractor (Hohmann), and the inferior neck is protected with a blunt-tipped retractor (Aufranc). As determined from a preoperative planning, the distance from the lesser trochanter to the level of the neck osteotomy is marked with the electrocautery.

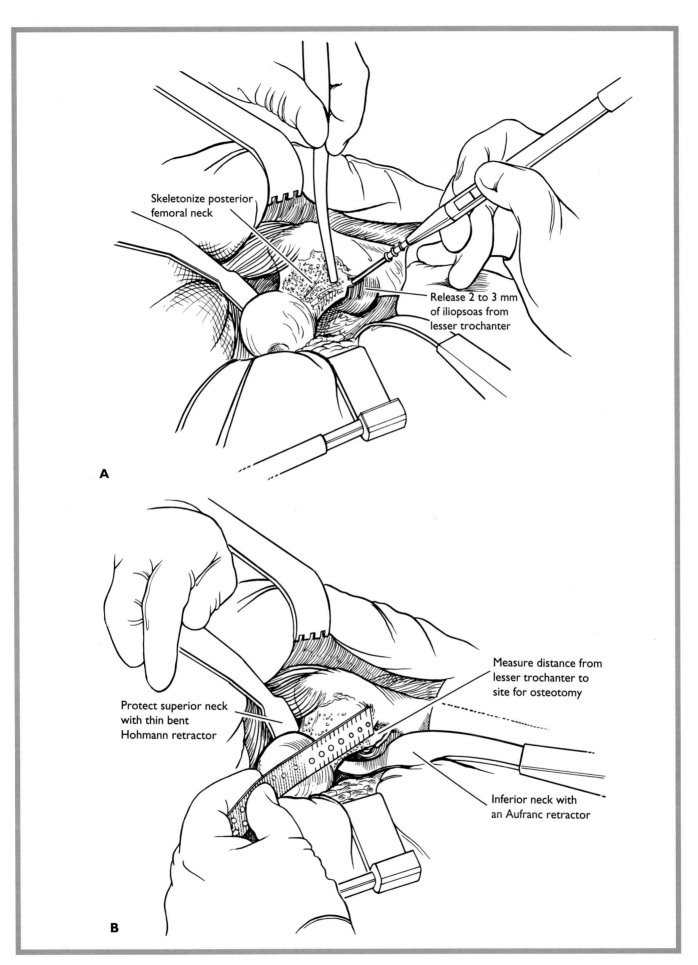

Skeletonize posterior femoral neck

Release 2 to 3 mm of iliopsoas from lesser trochanter

A

Protect superior neck with thin bent Hohmann retractor

Measure distance from lesser trochanter to site for osteotomy

Inferior neck with an Aufranc retractor

B

Femoral Neck Osteotomy

A.

The angle of the cut is marked using a trial prosthesis. The level of the cut should be double checked by matching the center of rotation of the femoral head to the center of rotation of the prosthetic head.

B.

The femoral neck is cut using a power operated oscillating saw. Care should be taken to avoid inadvertent osteotomy of either the greater trochanter or the distal portion of the femoral neck, which may predispose to fracture. The femoral head is removed from the operative field. The femoral retractors are now removed, and the leg is allowed to return to an extended and neutral rotation position.

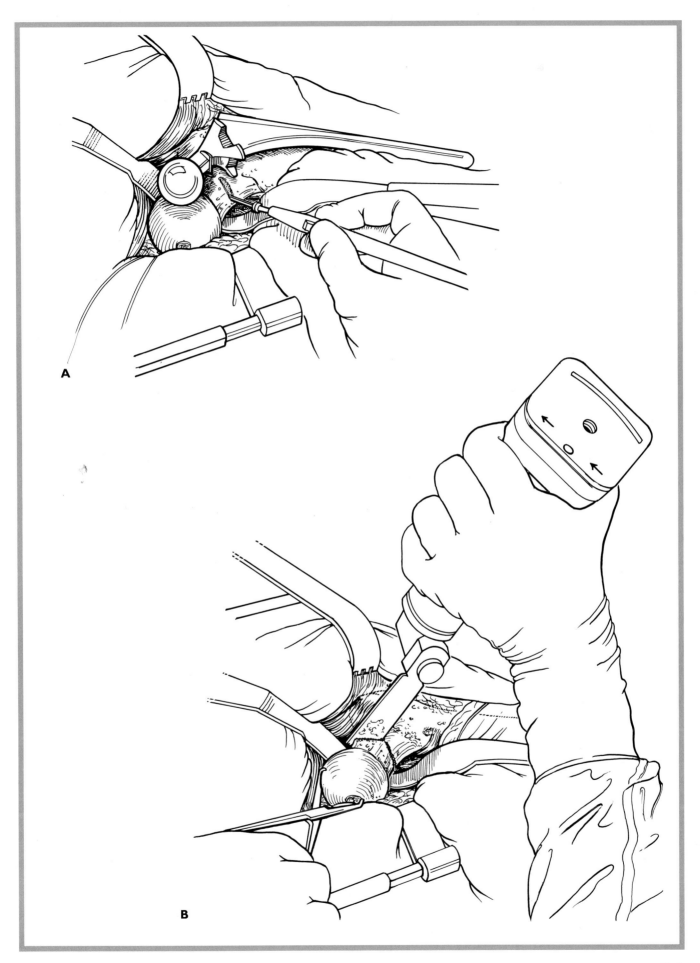

A

B

4

Acetabular Exposure and Reaming

Acetabular Exposure

A.

Anterior: A curved pointed retractor (Hohmann—"C") is placed over the anterior acetabular lips intracapsularly. This is retracted forward (anterior).

B.

Superior: A smooth Steinmann pin is used to gently retract the gluteus maximus and medius musculature superiorly. This is impacted into the ilium.

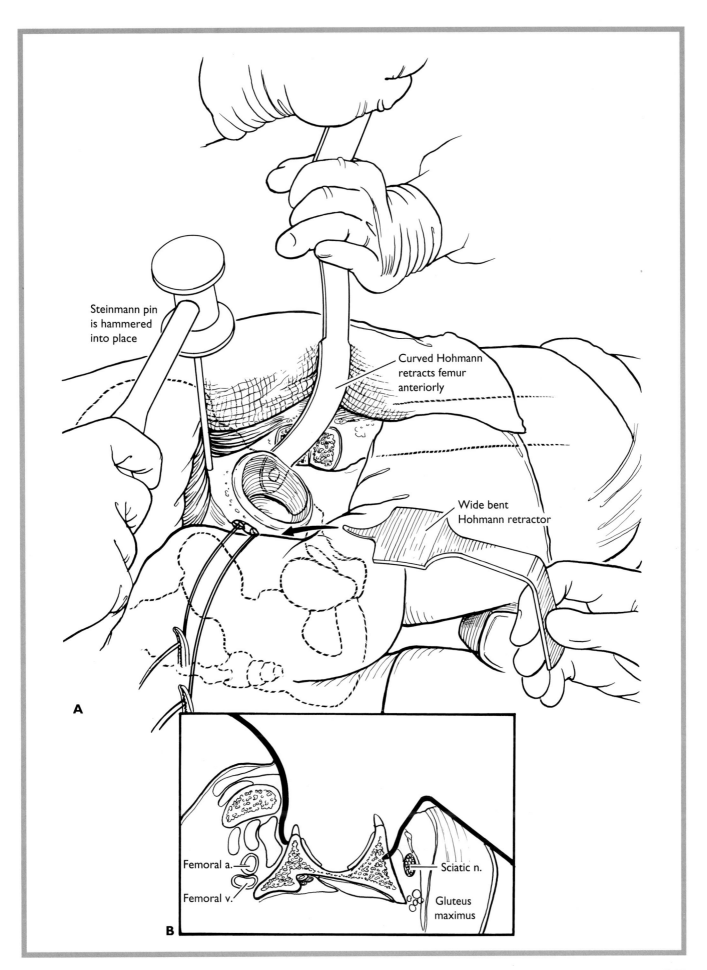

Steinmann pin is hammered into place

Curved Hohmann retracts femur anteriorly

Wide bent Hohmann retractor

A

B

Femoral a.

Femoral v.

Sciatic n.

Gluteus maximus

35

C.

Posterior: A broad angled, sharply pointed retractor is then impacted into the ischium intracapsularly to provide posterior exposure. A broad blunt-tipped retractor (Aufranc) is placed just outside the inferior capsular cut in the obturator foramen. This should be held by an assistant.

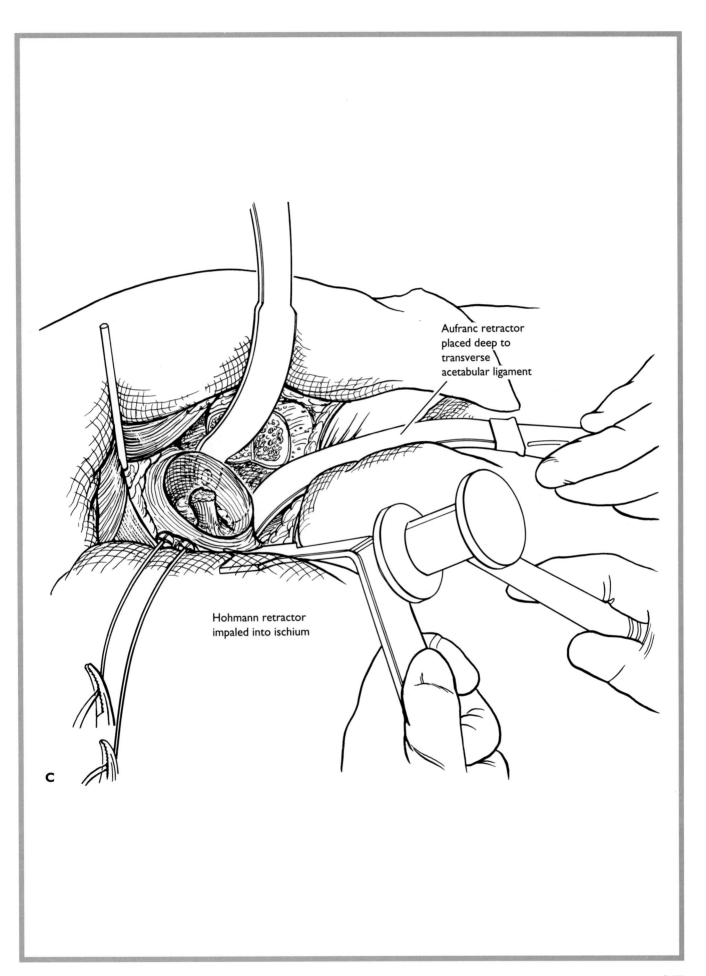

Aufranc retractor
placed deep to
transverse
acetabular ligament

Hohmann retractor
impaled into ischium

C

Difficult Acetabular Exposure

A.

If the exposure is still suboptimal, several maneuvers will help. The reflected head of the rectus femoris can be released superiorly and anteriorly just in front of the Steinmann pin using electrocautery.

B.

There is often residual superior capsule that will prevent anterior displacement of the femur. Complete relief of the superior capsule is essential for adequate exposure. Further release of the inferior capsule will also allow mobilization of the femur.

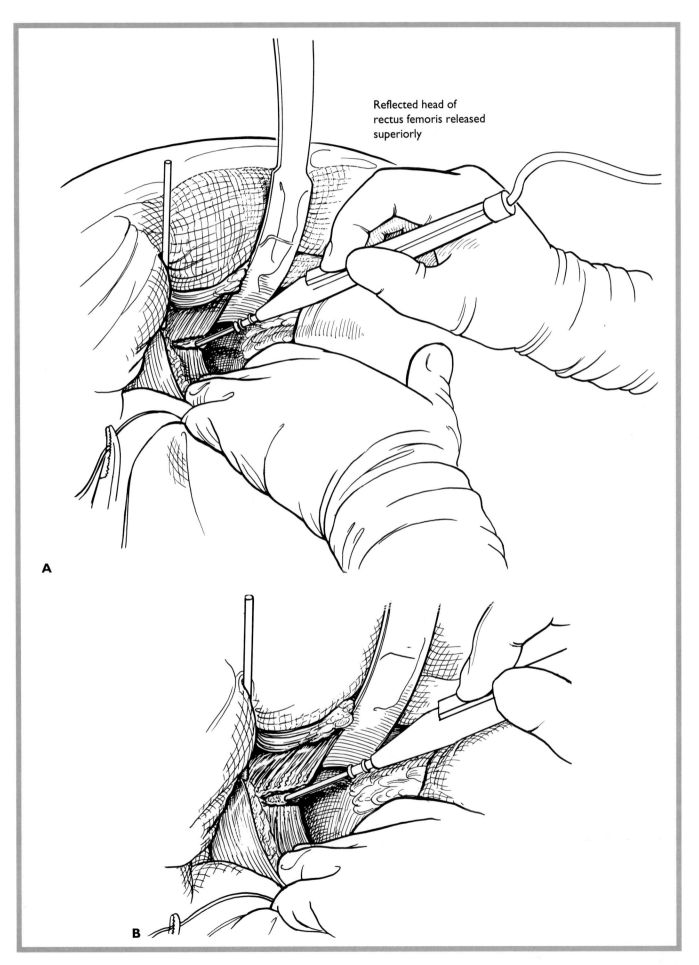

Reflected head of
rectus femoris released
superiorly

A

B

39

Acetabular Preparation

The labrum and pulvinar are excised with the use of the rongeur and electrocautery. The presence of medial osteophyte often obscures the pulvinar. The osteophyte should be removed with either a reamer, curette, or gouge. It is essential to adequately identify the true medial wall of the acetabulum.

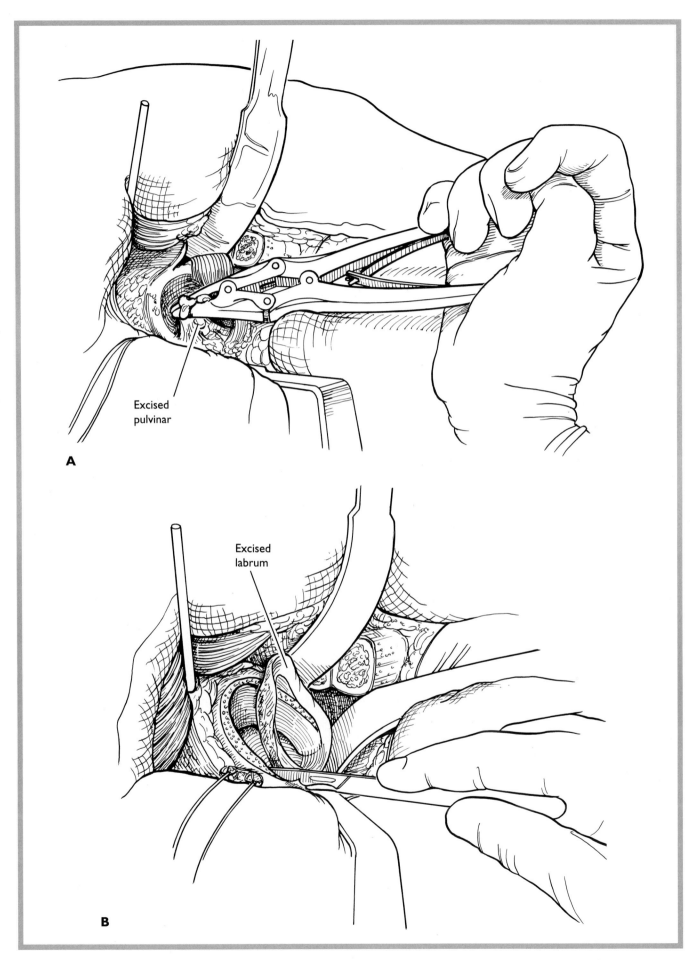

Excised
pulvinar

A

Excised
labrum

B

Preparation for Acetabular Reaming

At this point the Aufranc retractor should be placed deep to the transverse acetabular ligament and inside the joint capsule to reveal the inferomedial border of the true acetabulum ("teardrop"). Battery-powered grater-type reamers should be used to first remove all remnants of medial osteophyte. The radius of curvature of the dome should match that of the lateral cortex of the medial wall.

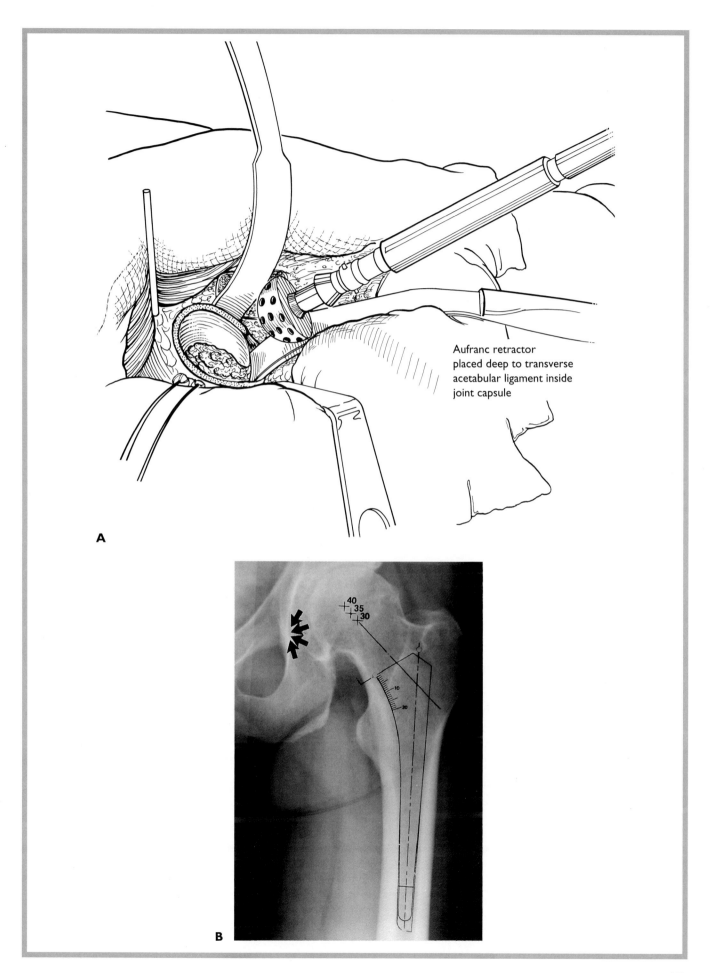

A

Aufranc retractor
placed deep to transverse
acetabular ligament inside
joint capsule

B

Acetabular Reaming

Progressively larger power reamers should be used to expand the acetabulum until the subchondral plate of the dome begins to reveal cancellous bone. The plate should not be removed entirely as it provides strength. Continual monitoring of anterior and posterior walls is necessary to prevent them from becoming thin. *The lateral cortex of the medial wall must not be violated.*

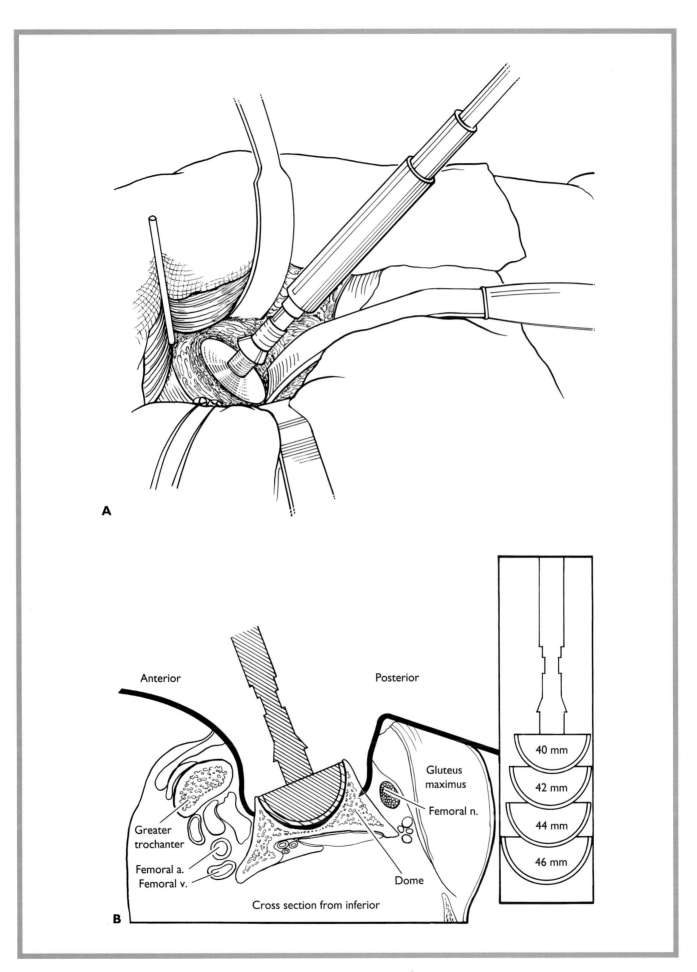

A

B

Anterior

Posterior

Greater
trochanter

Femoral a.
Femoral v.

Gluteus
maximus

Femoral n.

Dome

Cross section from inferior

40 mm

42 mm

44 mm

46 mm

Acetabular Sizing

The proper component will allow approximately 3 cm of cement to surround it yet still be contained within the bony confines. The use of acetabular components with pods allows uniform cement to mantle around the implant. Insufficient cement mantle may lead to early component failure.

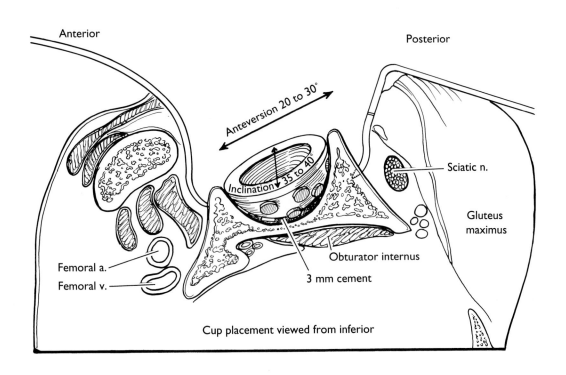

Anterior

Posterior

Anteversion 20 to 30°

Inclination 35 to 40°

Sciatic n.

Gluteus maximus

Obturator internus

Femoral a.

Femoral v.

3 mm cement

Cup placement viewed from inferior

47

5

Placement of Acetabular Component

Acetabular Positioning

A.

When using a posterior approach, acetabular inclination of 30 to 40 degrees and anteversion of 15 to 25 degrees are optimal. Because over 90 percent of dislocations following the posterior approach are posterior in nature, additional acetabular anteversion affords greater hip stability.

Landmarks for acetabular inclination are the posterior and superior iliac spines. Preoperatively, a line should be positioned through the iliac spines perpendicular to the floor. In this way, the floor can be used as a reference point during cup insertion.

B.

Anteversion can be determined by referencing the highest point of the crest of the ilium, the anterior superior iliac spine and the posterior superior iliac spine. The bisecting line of this triangle will approximate neutral version. In general, when acetabular anatomy is normal, intrinsic anteversion is about 10 to 15 degrees.

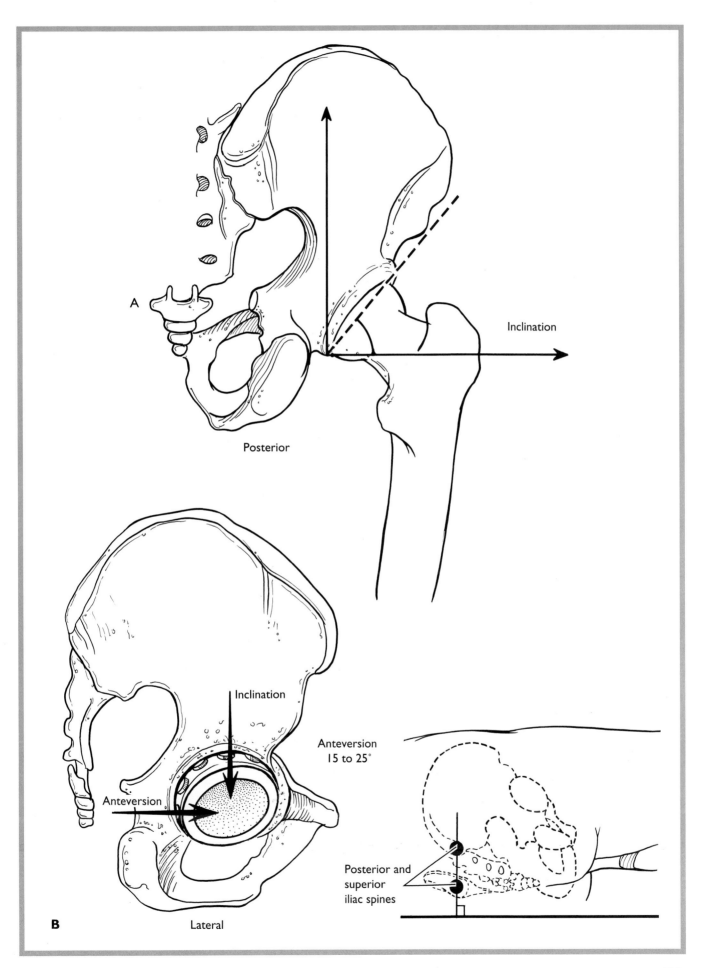

A

Inclination

Posterior

Inclination

Anteversion
15 to 25°

Anteversion

B

Lateral

Posterior and
superior
iliac spines

51

Acetabular Bed Preparation

A.

A Cobb gouge or a curette is used to make large (1 cm in diameter) fixation holes in the pubis and ischium.

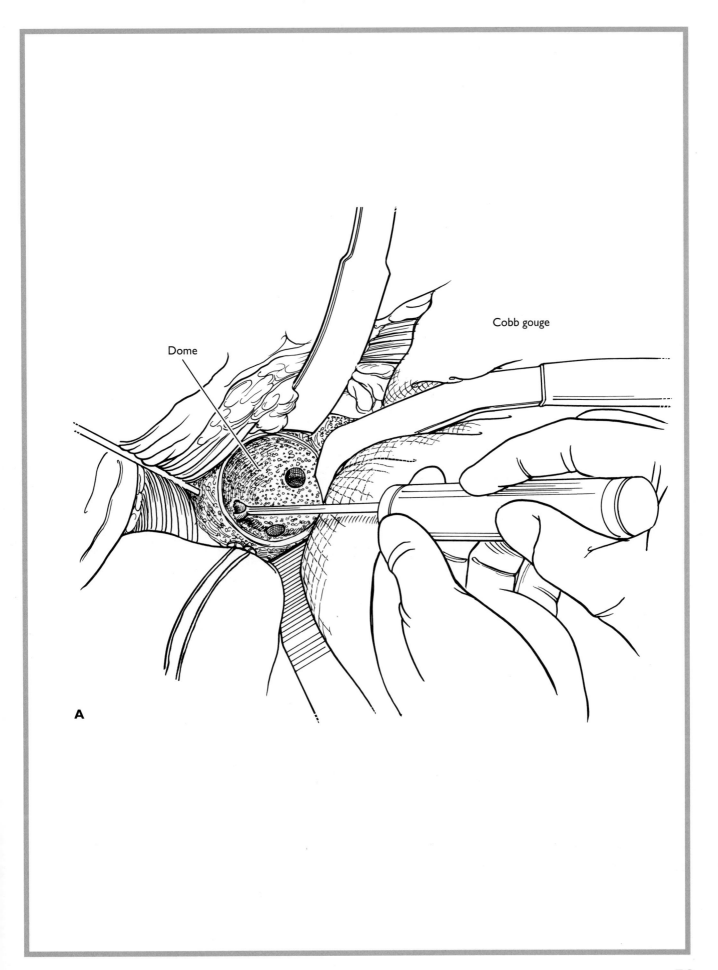

Dome

Cobb gouge

A

B.

A Midas Rex is used to make smaller (3 mm in diameter) fixation holes
in the dome portion of the ilium.

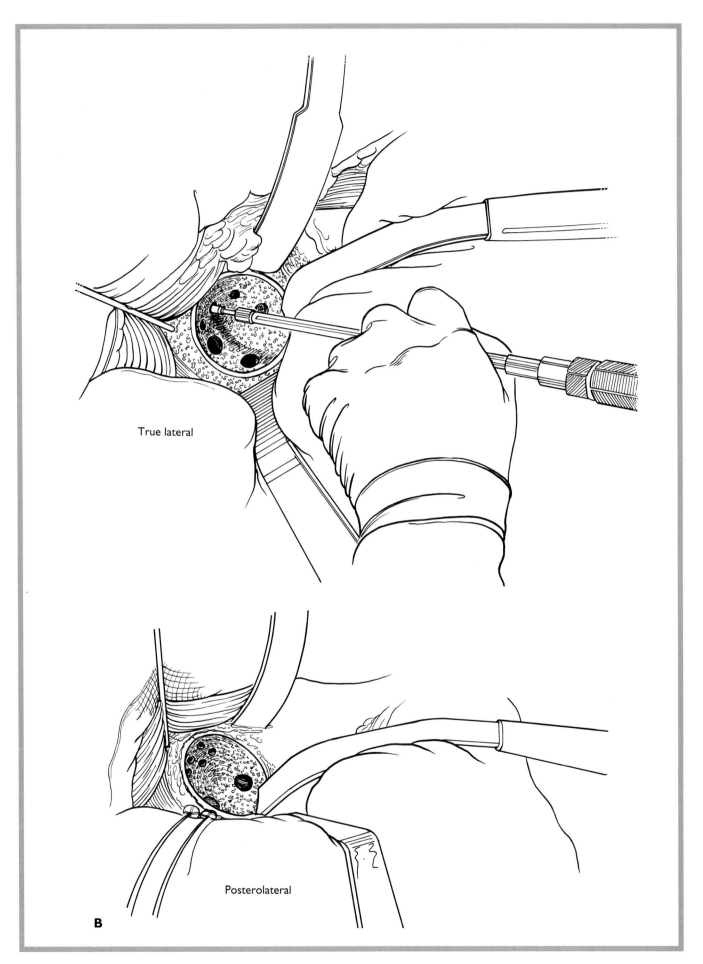

True lateral

Posterolateral

B

C.

The bony bed is irrigated with pulsatile lavage and dried with a lap sponge. The bed is pressurized with a second dry lap sponge to keep it dry while the cement is being prepared. Hypotensive anesthesia helps maintain a dry acetabular bed for improved bone cement interdigitation.

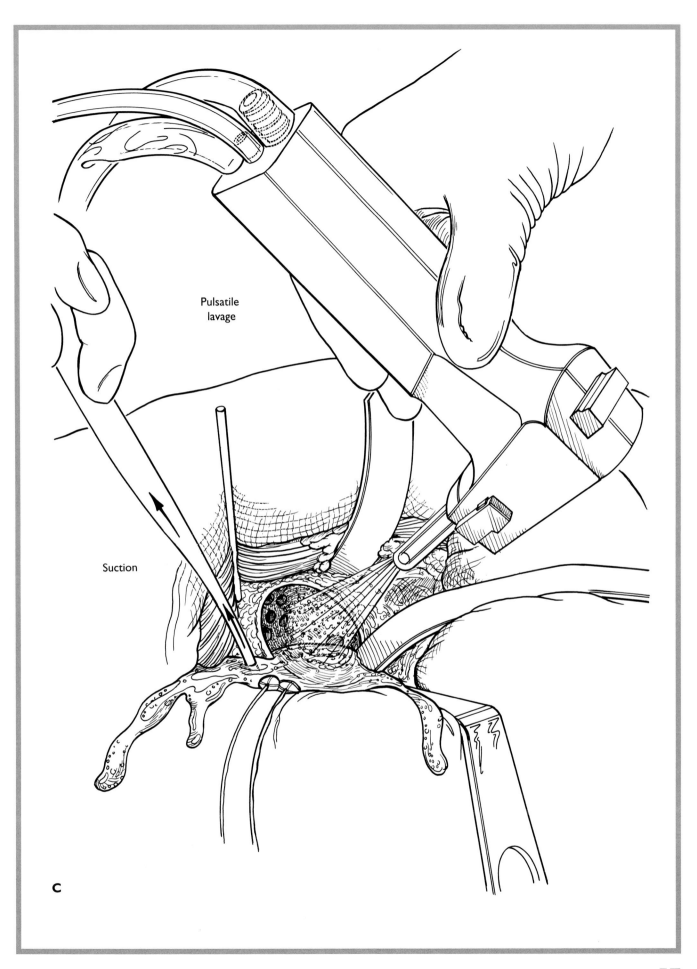

Pulsatile
lavage

Suction

C

Cement Preparation

A.

It is recommended that two large packages (80 g total) of polymethyl-methacrylate are used for fixation of acetabular components that are 40 mm or larger. Smaller diameter components may only require one package of polymethylmethacrylate. The cement should be vacuum mixed or centrifuged in order to minimize voids and thus improve fatigue properties.

B.

The packing used to keep the acetabular bed dry is removed, and the cement is rounded to fit the size of the acetabular bed.

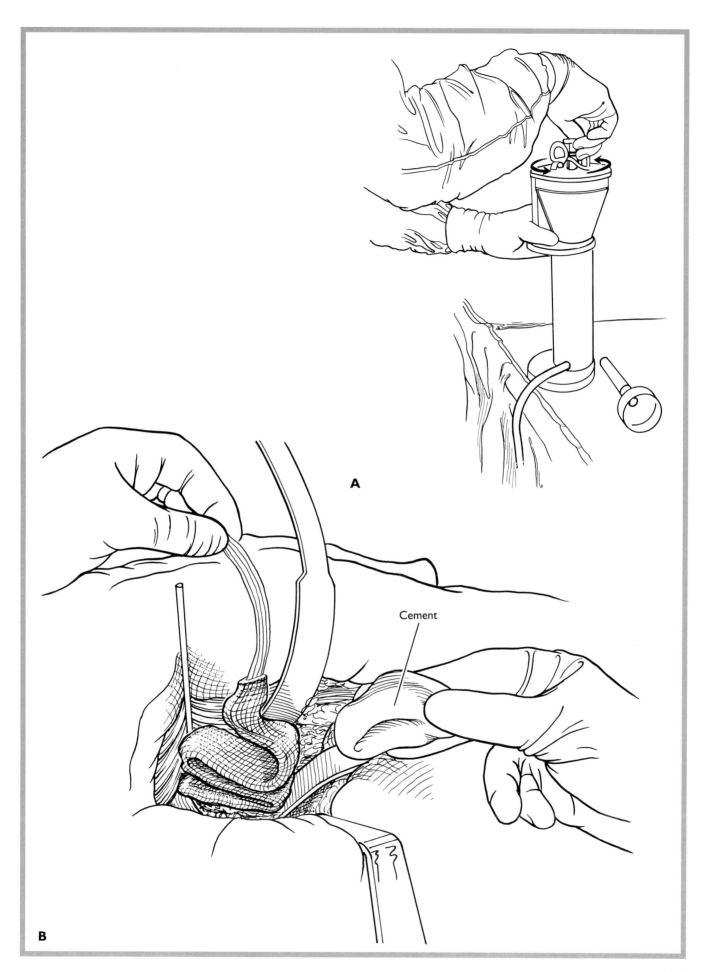

A

Cement

B

59

Cement Insertion

A.

The cement is handled in the doughy phase. It is placed en masse in the acetabulum.

B.

The cement is pressurized with a bulb syringe that effectively occludes egress of cement.

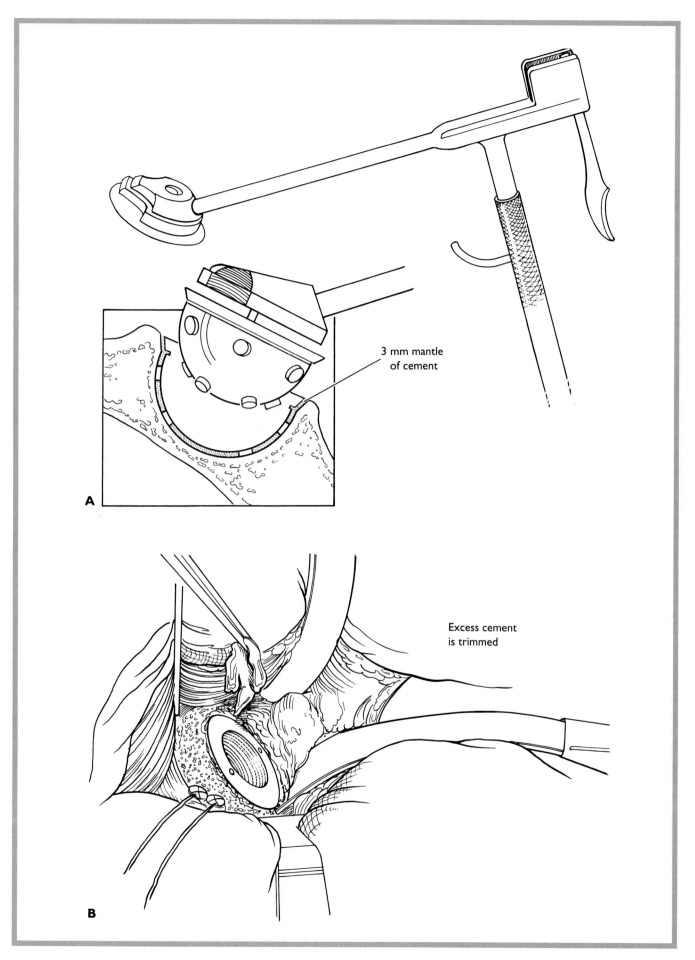

3 mm mantle
of cement

A

Excess cement
is trimmed

B

Socket Insertion

A.

The acetabular insertion guide should be oriented to allow 40 degrees of vertical inclination and approximately 20 degrees of anteversion period. Care should be taken not to "bottom-out" the acetabular component, thus leading to an excessively thin cement mantle supporting the component period. A 3 mm mantle of cement is optimal. The use of acetabular components with acrylic pods helps to result in this uniform cement mantle. Pressure should be maintained on the component until the cement has fully polymerized.

B.

At this time, excess cement is trimmed away from the component.

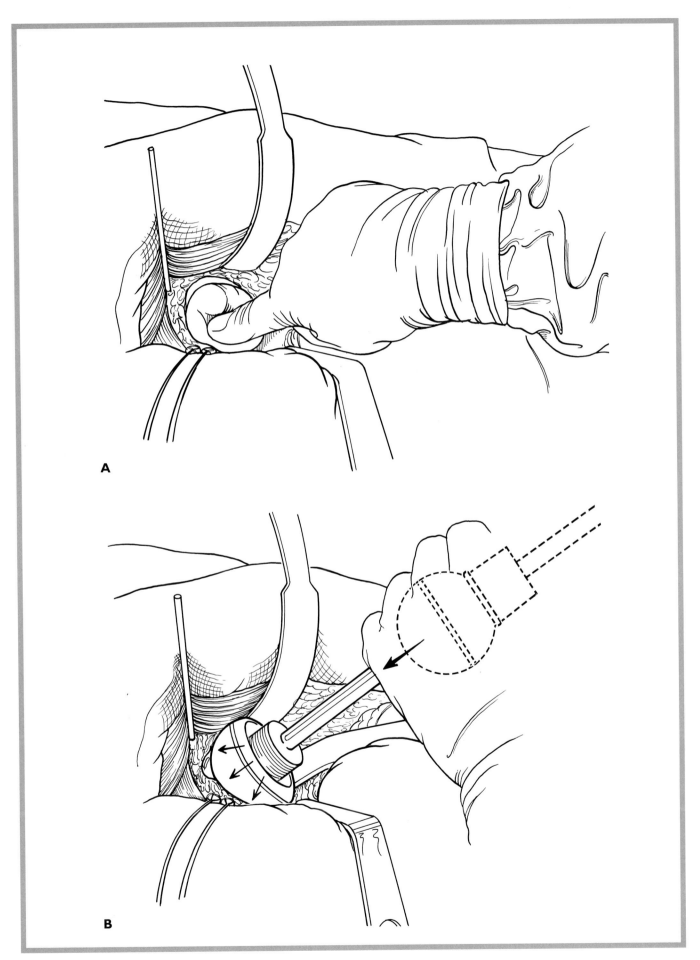

A

B

Wound Care

A.

Polyethylene lavage is used to irrigate the wound with an antibiotic solution. The wound drapes should be kept moist throughout the procedure.

B.

A moist sponge is placed over the acetabular component as a protective measure during femoral preparation.

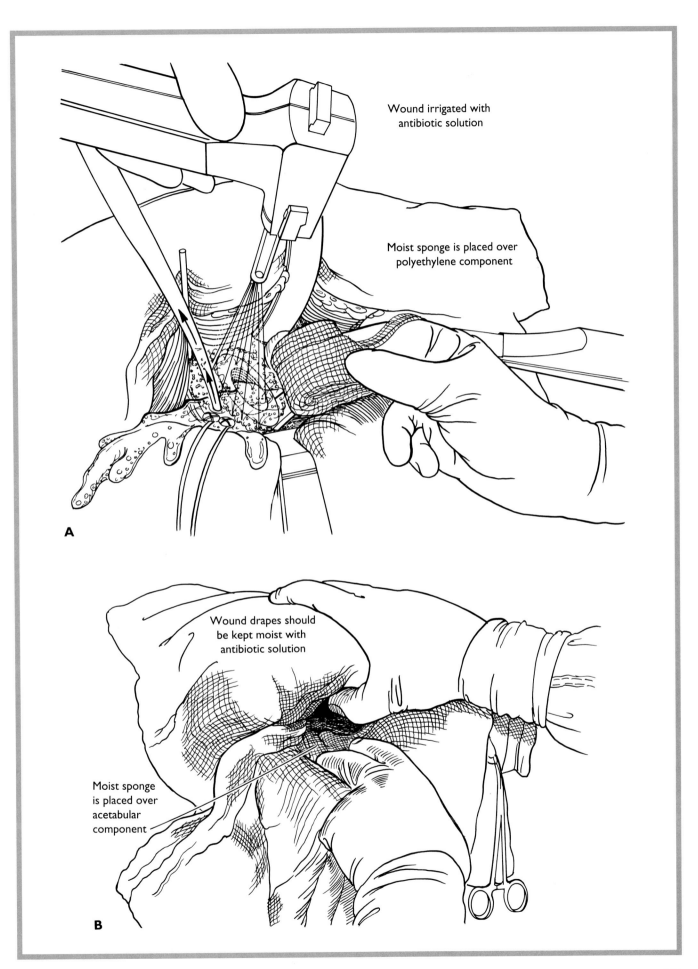

Wound irrigated with antibiotic solution

Moist sponge is placed over polyethylene component

A

Wound drapes should be kept moist with antibiotic solution

Moist sponge is placed over acetabular component

B

6

Femoral Shaft Exposure and Reaming

Femoral Preparation

A.

When employing the posterolateral approach, at this point, the femur is flexed to 90 degrees and internally rotated to 90 degrees with the proximal end of the femur delivered into the wound.

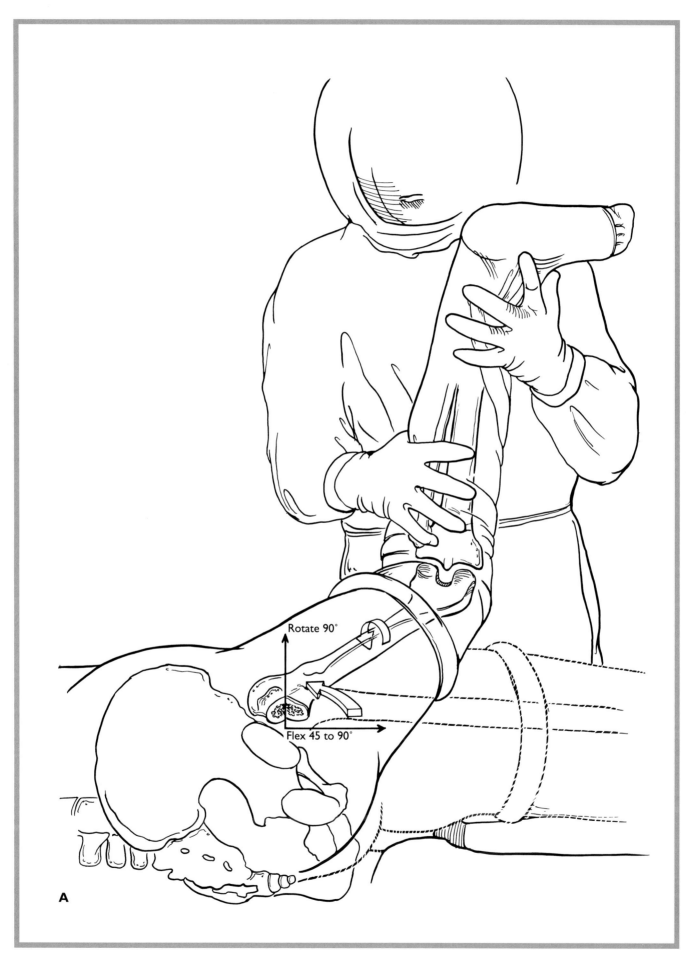

A

B.

An example of a proximal femoral retractor used during femoral preparation.

C.

The proximal femoral retractor is placed under the neck of the femur, which is then levered out of the wound. This will provide access to the femoral canal.

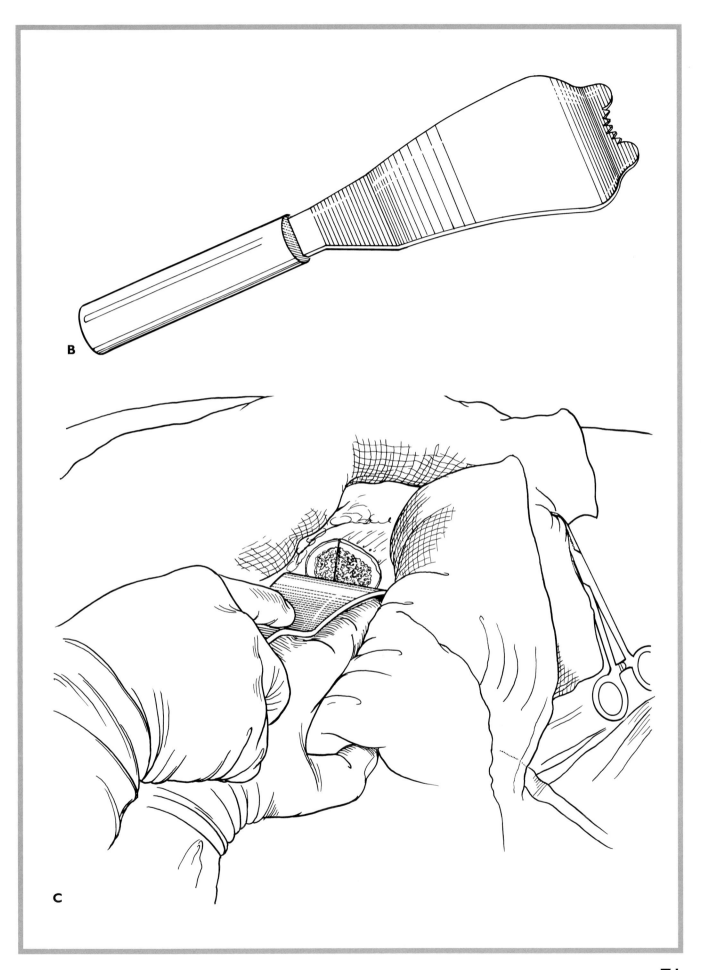

B

C

71

D.

A blunt retractor (Aufranc) is placed under the medial edge of the proximal femoral retractor to clear the posterior aspect of the upper part of the femur from the adjacent soft tissue.

E.

A thin bent retractor (Hohmann) is placed deep to the abductor musculature and over the tip of the greater trochanter to expose the junction between the femoral neck and the greater trochanter.

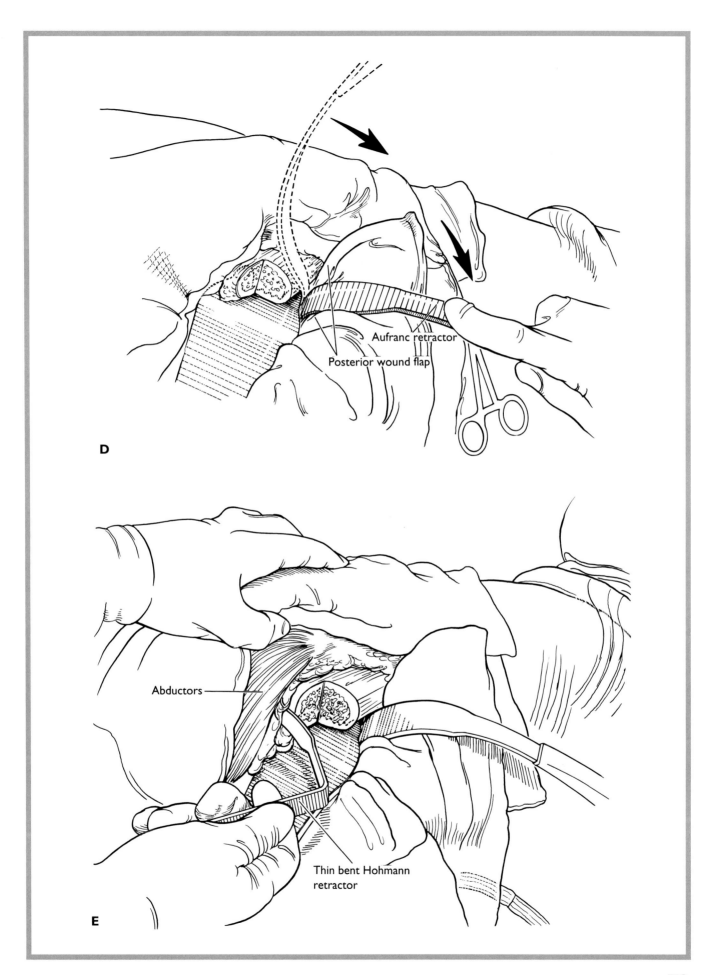

Aufranc retractor

Posterior wound flap

D

Abductors

Thin bent Hohmann
retractor

E

F.

This retractor protects the abductor musculature during femoral preparation.

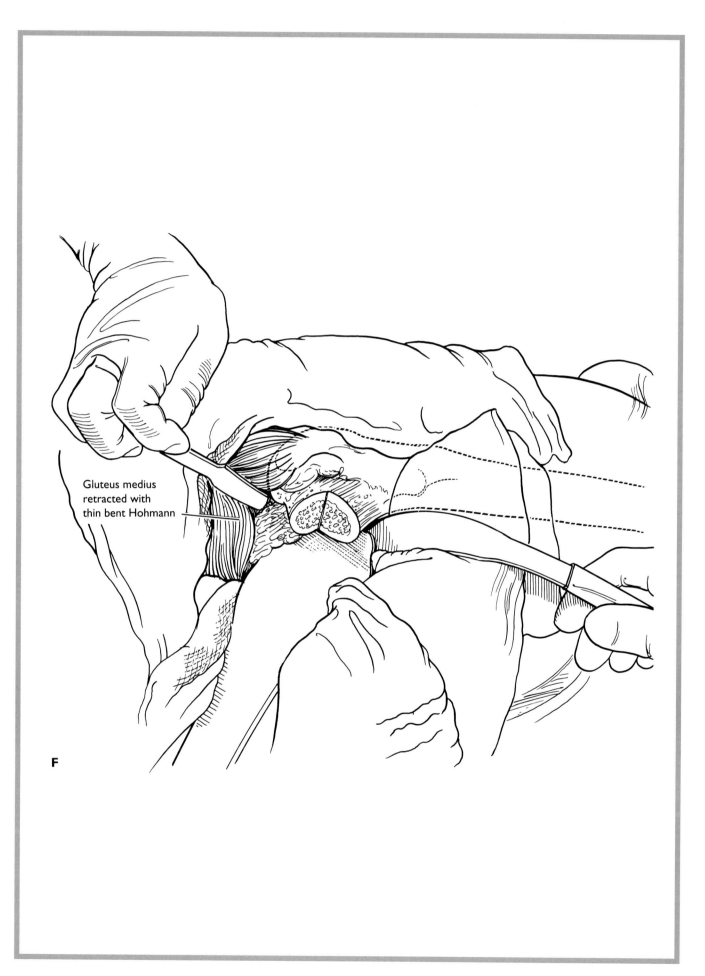

Gluteus medius
retracted with
thin bent Hohmann

F

Femoral Canal Preparation

A.

Remnants of capsule and external rotators that can obscure the junction between femoral neck and trochanter are excised for complete exposure of the lateral neck.

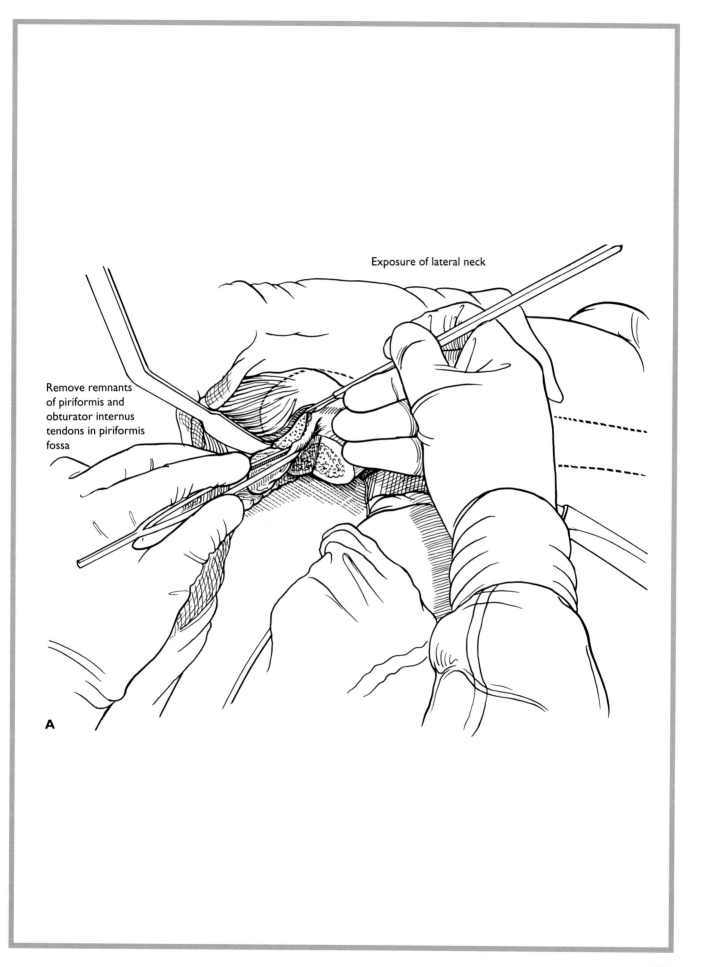

Exposure of lateral neck

Remove remnants
of piriformis and
obturator internus
tendons in piriformis
fossa

A

B.

The remnant of the femoral neck is now trimmed to the base of the greater trochanter. This can be performed with the use of a rongeur, an osteotome, or a gouge.

C.

Resection of the lateral neck permits direct visualization and allows access directly into the femoral canal. Failure to adequately remove the remaining portion of femoral neck can compromise instrumentation of the femoral canal and increase the risk of femoral cortical perforation.

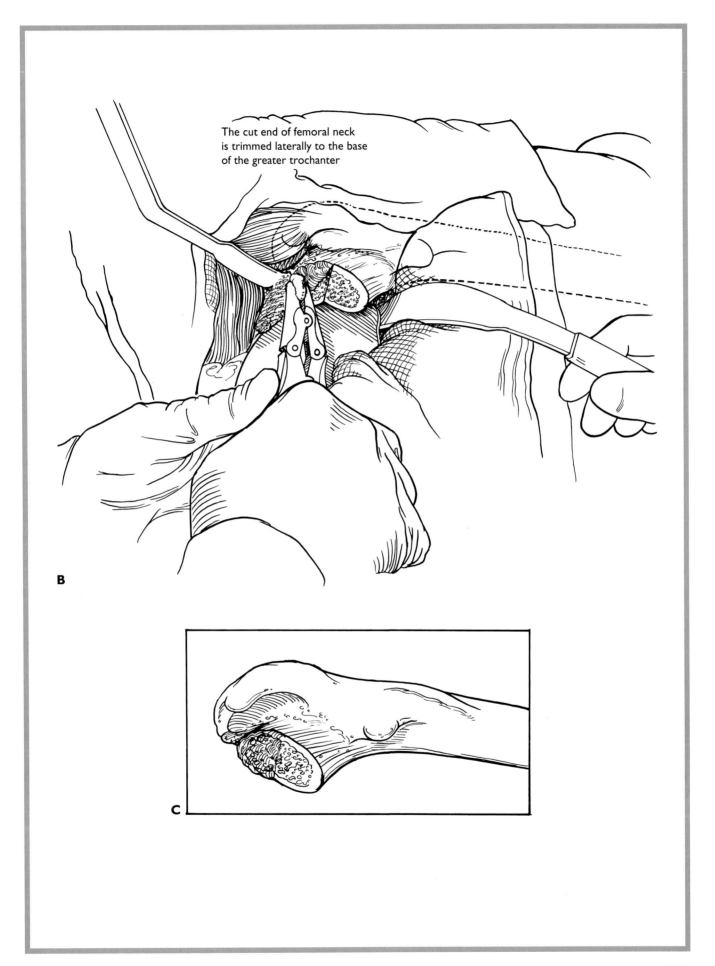

The cut end of femoral neck
is trimmed laterally to the base
of the greater trochanter

B

C

Femoral Canal Reaming

A.

An end-cutting hand-held reamer is used to access the femoral canal.

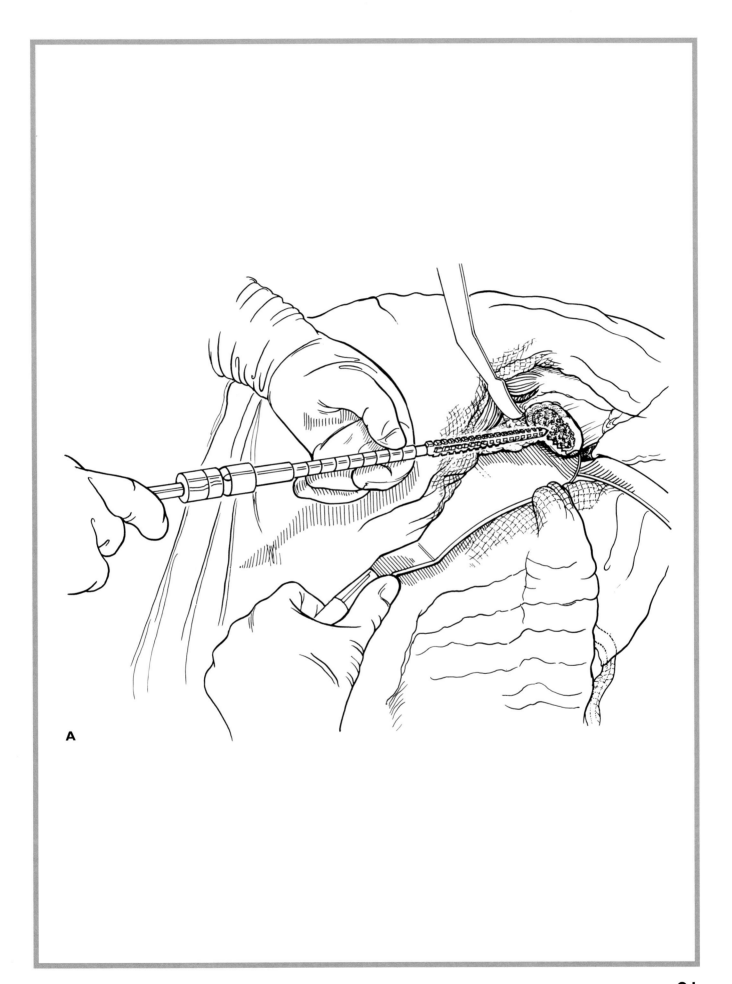

A

B.

The reamer should be started laterally in the neck to avoid the need for excessive varus direction to "find" the canal.

C.

A closer view more clearly defines placement.

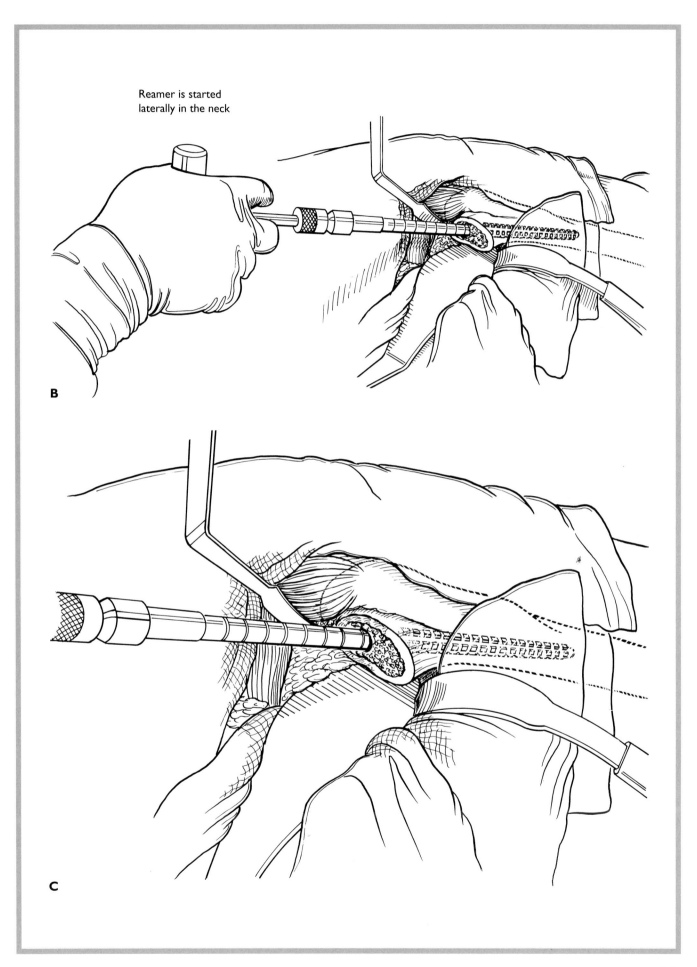

Reamer is started
laterally in the neck

B

C

Femoral Canal Enlargement

The canal is enlarged sequentially with truncated conical hand or power driven reamers to the appropriate size as estimated preoperatively. Reaming should stop and the stem should be downsized if hard endosteal bone or cortical contact is encountered prior to the templated size.

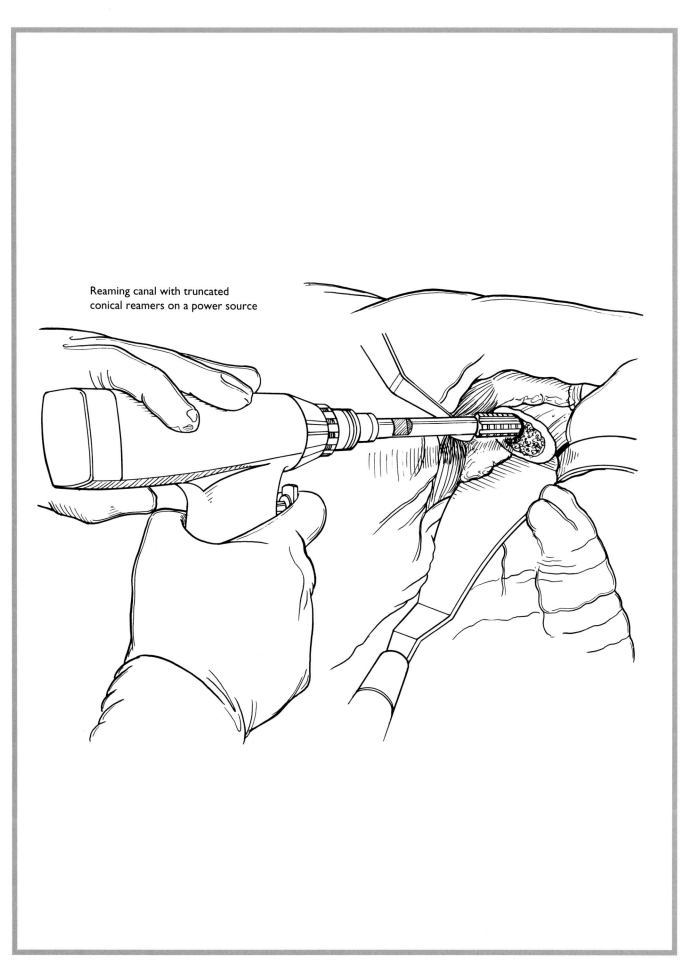

Reaming canal with truncated
conical reamers on a power source

Broach Trials

Broaches that match the size and shape of the femoral components are used sequentially to enlarge and shape the metaphyseal region so that it will accommodate the desired size stem. These wedge-like broaches should be impacted gently to avoid fracturing the femur.

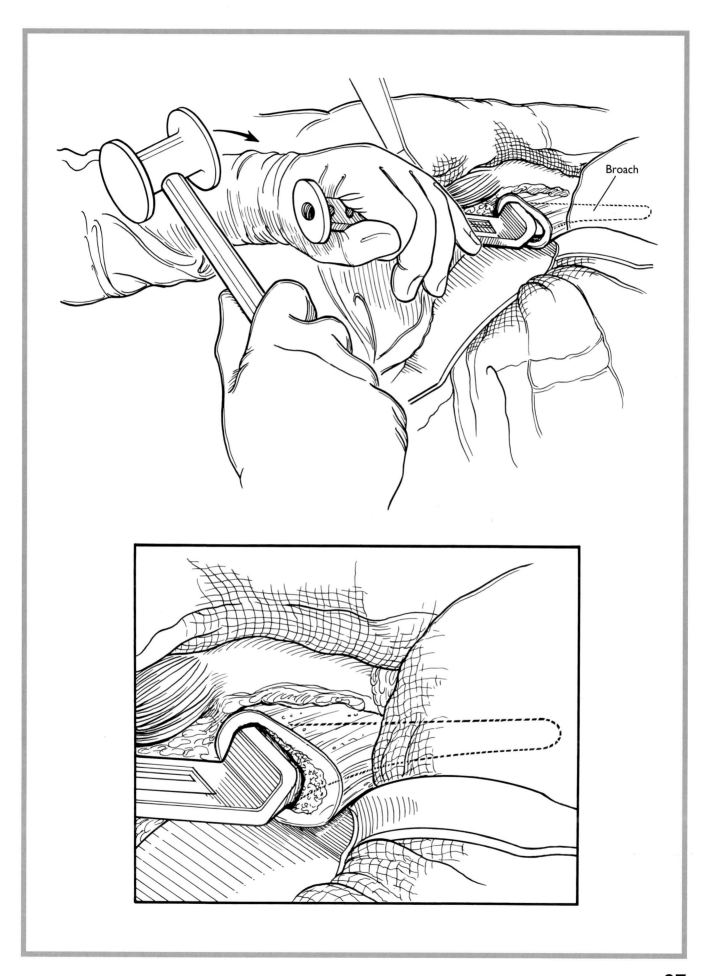

Broach

Broach and Cancellous Bone Removal

A.

The broach is gently removed from the proximal femur in the line that it was inserted to prevent fracture.

B.

Loose cancellous bone is removed from the proximal femur with a curette. This should be performed in a gentle manner to avoid removal of firmly fixed cancellous bone.

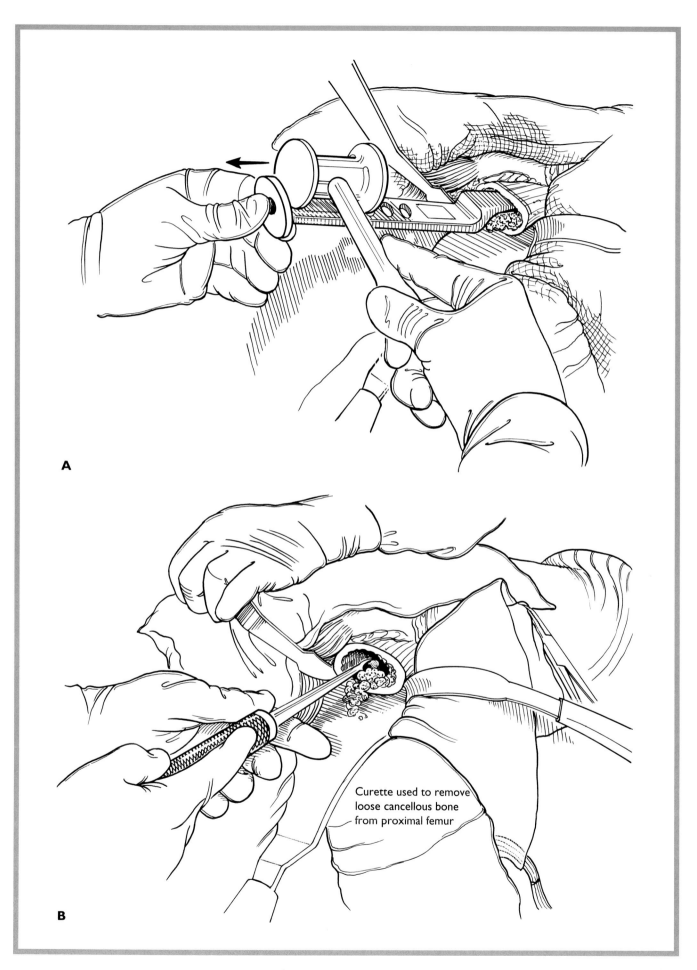

A

B

Curette used to remove
loose cancellous bone
from proximal femur

Trial Reduction

A.

Sample of trial femoral component.

B.

The trial femoral component is inserted with the appropriate head/neck assembly.

C.

At this point the lesser trochanter to center of rotation should be checked to assure proper restoration of leg length. Selection of an alternate head/neck assembly, or less commonly, further resection of the femoral neck may be necessary to reproduce the contralateral leg length.

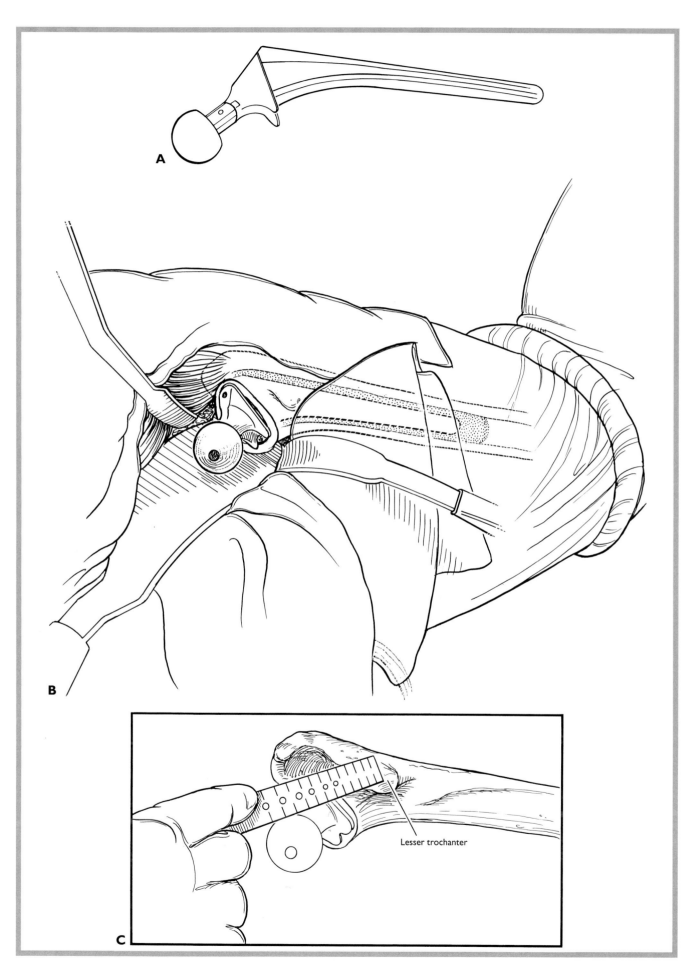

A

B

C

Lesser trochanter

D.

The hip is reduced.

E.

With the hip reduced, the patient is taken through a functional range-of-motion. Posterior stability of the hip is assessed by flexing and internally rotating the leg. Flexion of up to 90 degrees and internal rotation of up to 20 degrees with the hip stable is ideal. In addition, anterior instability must be assessed. This is performed by extending, abducting, and externally rotating the leg. The presence of osteophyte as well as a prominent trochanter can sometimes lead to bony impingement and be a source of instability. Removal of all prominent osteophyte can dramatically improve stability in some cases. Reassess component orientation of both the acetabular component as well as the femoral trial should instability persist. Lengthening of the leg by using a longer neck will often afford additional stability by increasing myofascial tension as well as increasing offset. Added offset will often eliminate the affect of bony impingement.

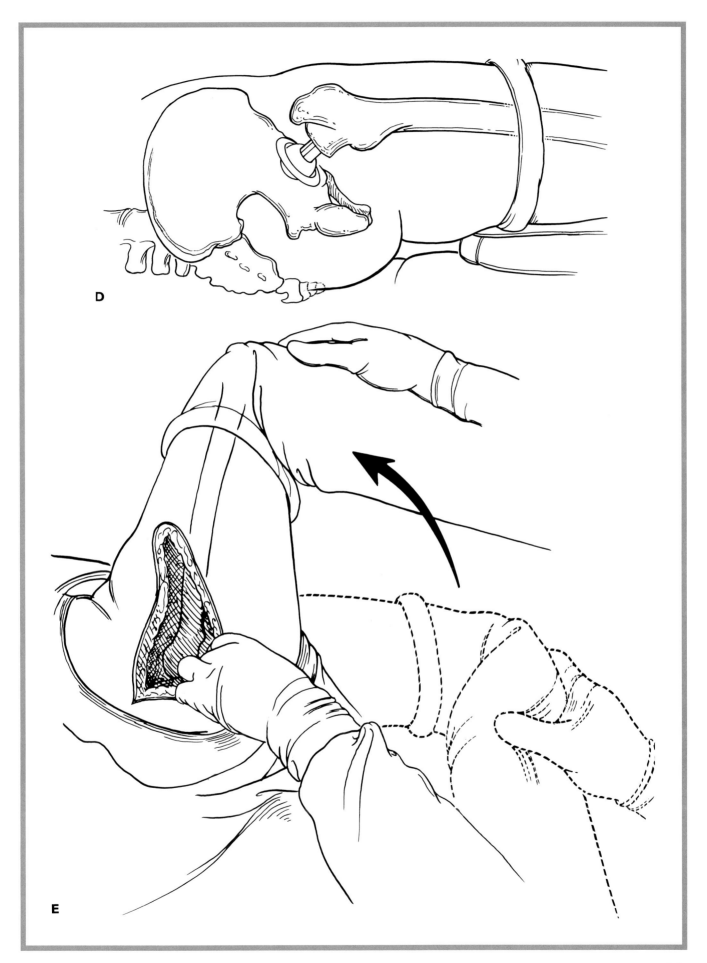

D

E

Wound Preparation

The hip is dislocated, and the trial femoral component is removed. The wound is irrigated, and the canal is curetted.

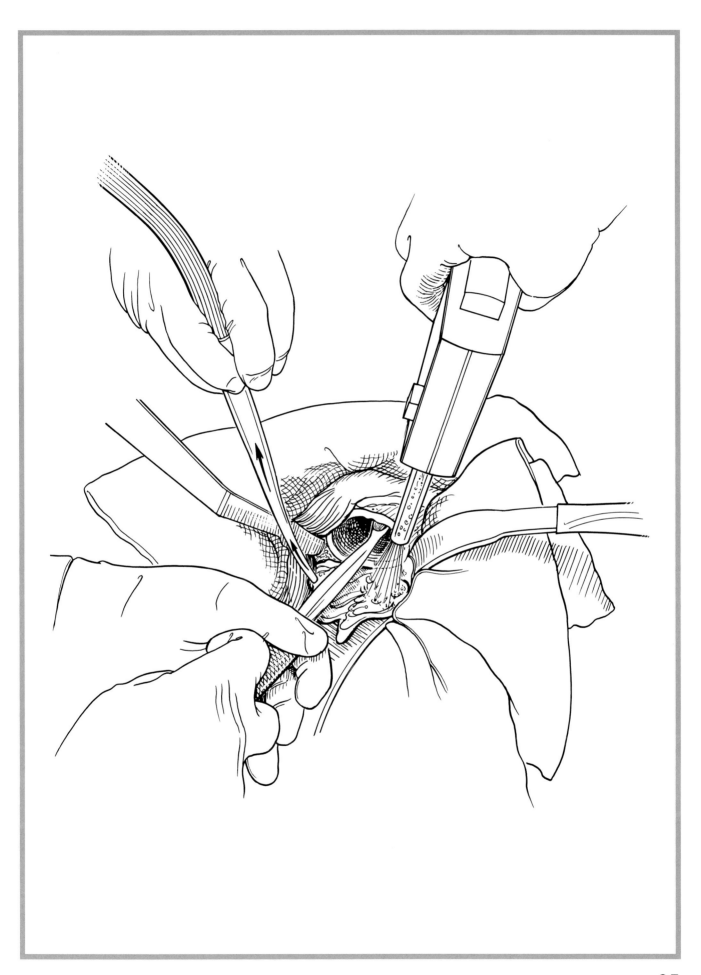

Femoral Canal Cement Preparation

A.

A polyethylene cement restrictor is inserted with a metal insertion rod.

B.

The shaft length of the femoral component is marked on the metal insertion rod to facilitate proper placement.

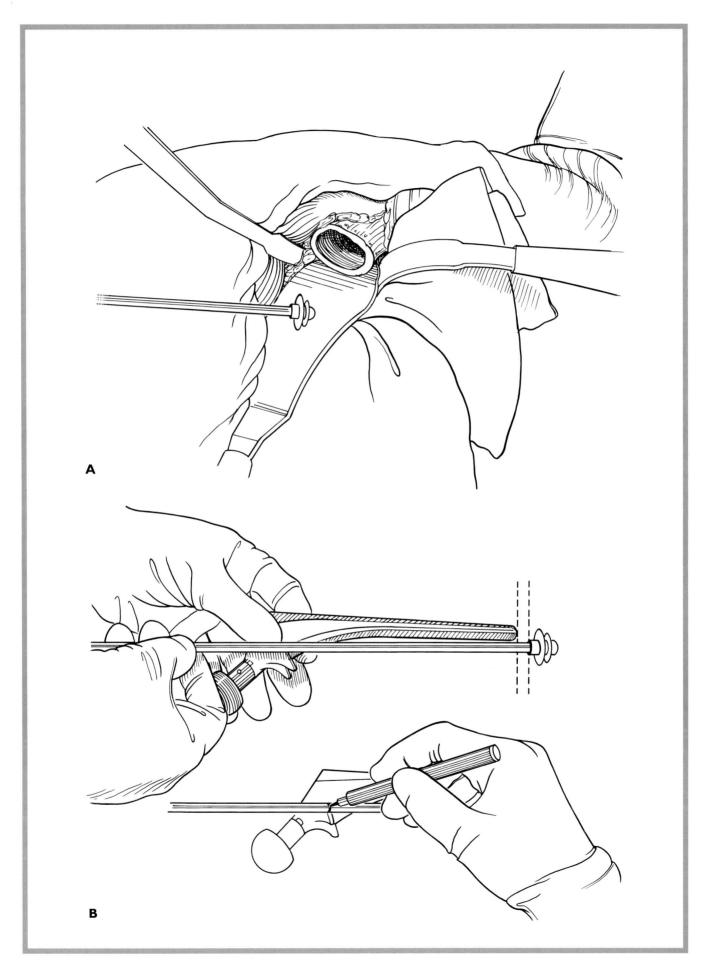

A

B

c.

The polyethylene cement restrictor is gently tapped into the cancellous bed at the end of the reamed canal. It should fit snugly 1 to 2 cm distal to the tip of the stem.

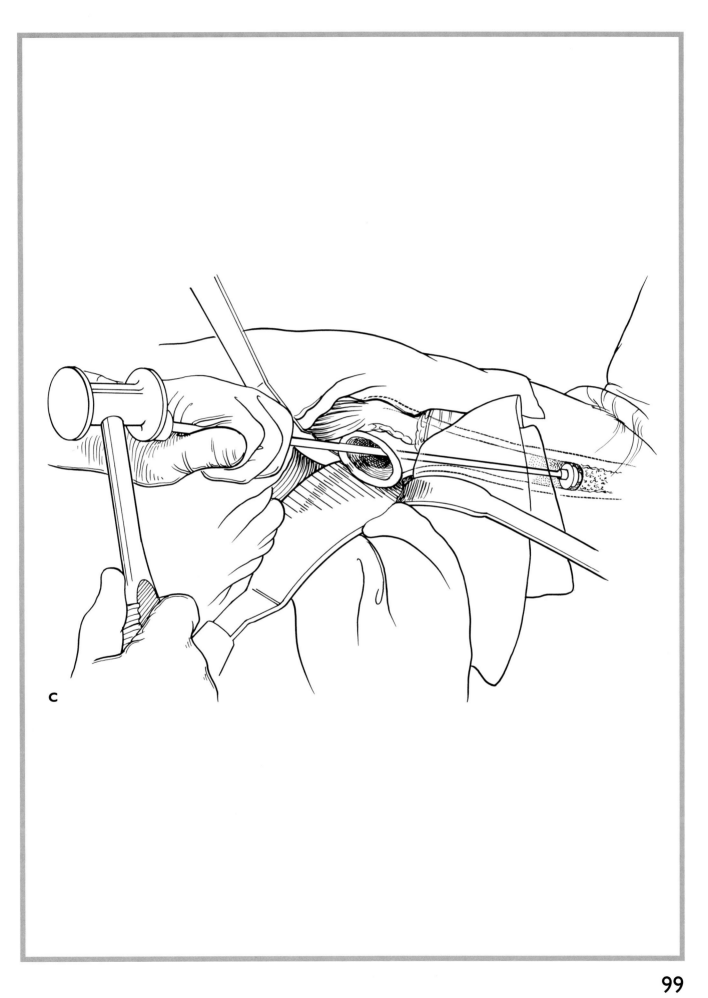

c

D.

A pulsatile lavage system is used to thoroughly clean the cancellous bone of the endosteum.

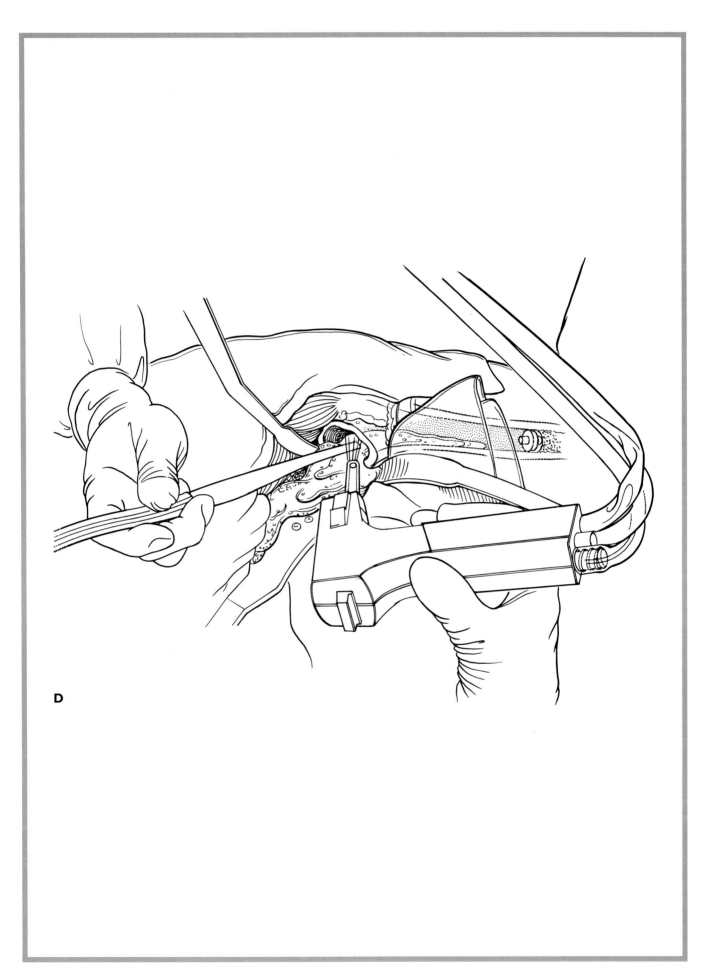

D

E.

As the cement is mixed, a vaginal packing is used to pack the canal tightly to keep the cancellous interstices dry.

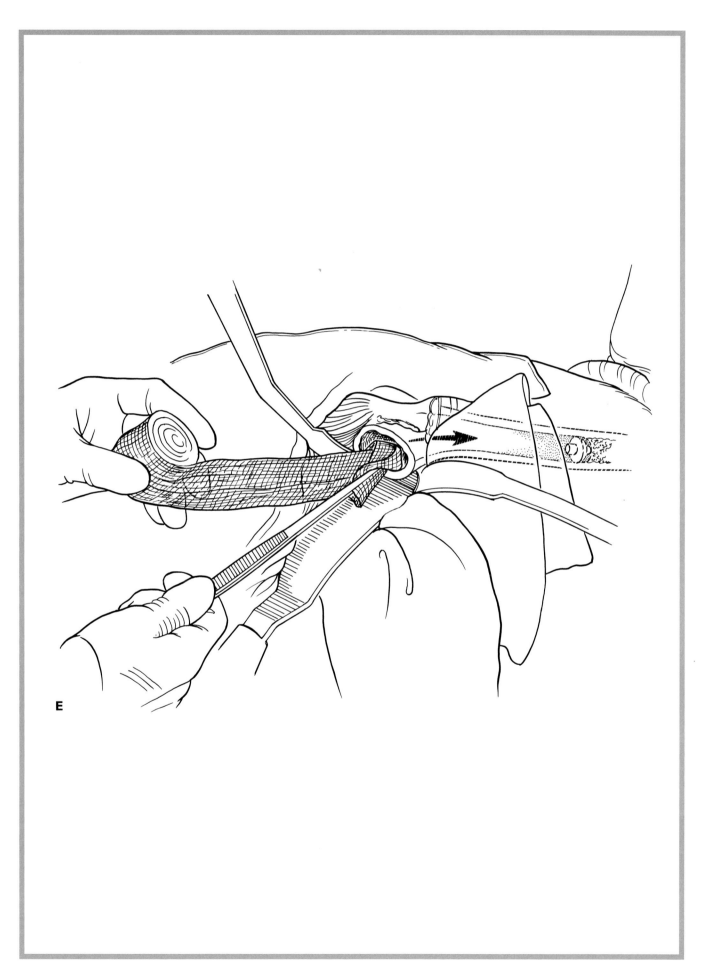

E

Cement Preparation

The cement is mixed in a vacuum-mixing system to minimize voids and increase fatigue strength.

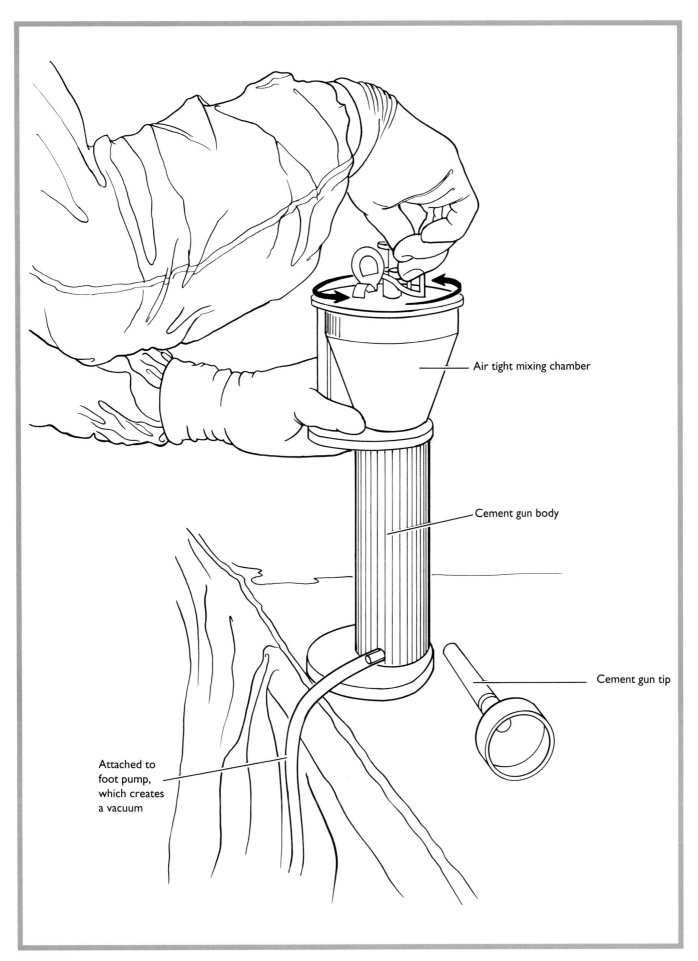

Air tight mixing chamber

Cement gun body

Cement gun tip

Attached to
foot pump,
which creates
a vacuum

Cement Placement

A.

When the cement is ready (early doughy phase), the packing is removed, and the canal is quickly aspirated.

B.

The canal is filled from distal to proximal using a cement gun.

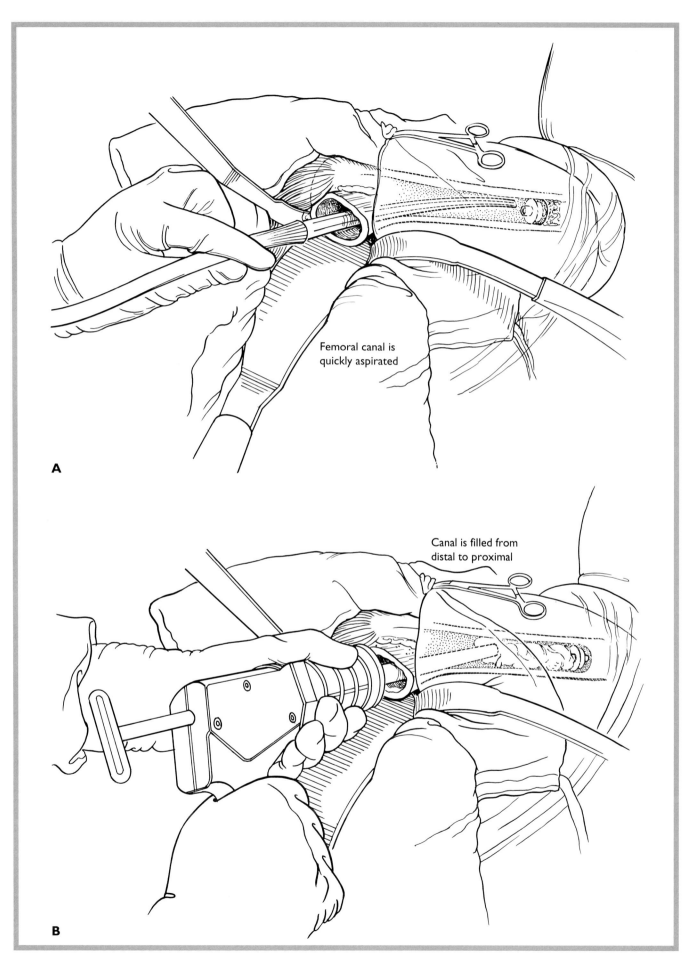

Femoral canal is
quickly aspirated

A

Canal is filled from
distal to proximal

B

107

Cement Pressurization

A.

The cement is pressurized manually using a specially adapted cement gun tip.

B.

Effective pressurization will result in the extrusion of blood and bone marrow from the nutrient foramen of the upper shaft of the femur. If the proximal pressuring instrument cannot obtain adequate seal during cementing, it is advised to use digital pressurization.

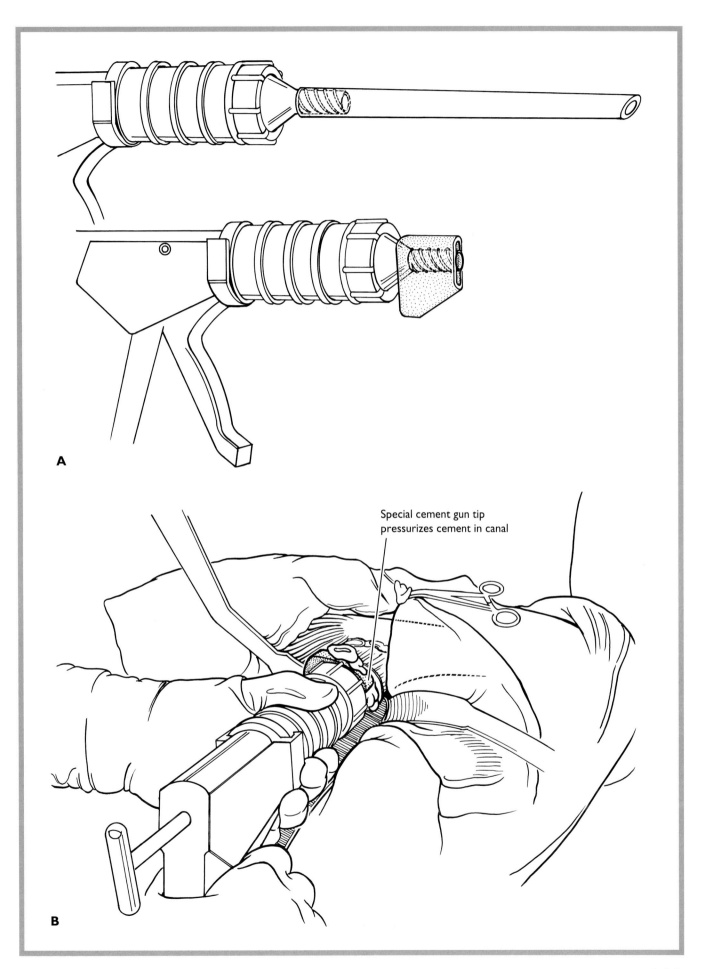

A

Special cement gun tip
pressurizes cement in canal

B

7

Placement of Femoral Component

Femoral Component Insertion

A.

The femoral component is inserted in neutral into the cement-field filled canal. The femoral component orientation should match that of the femoral neck. This will result in the femoral component with approximately 12 degrees of anteversion.

B.

Lateral view of anteversion of the femoral neck.

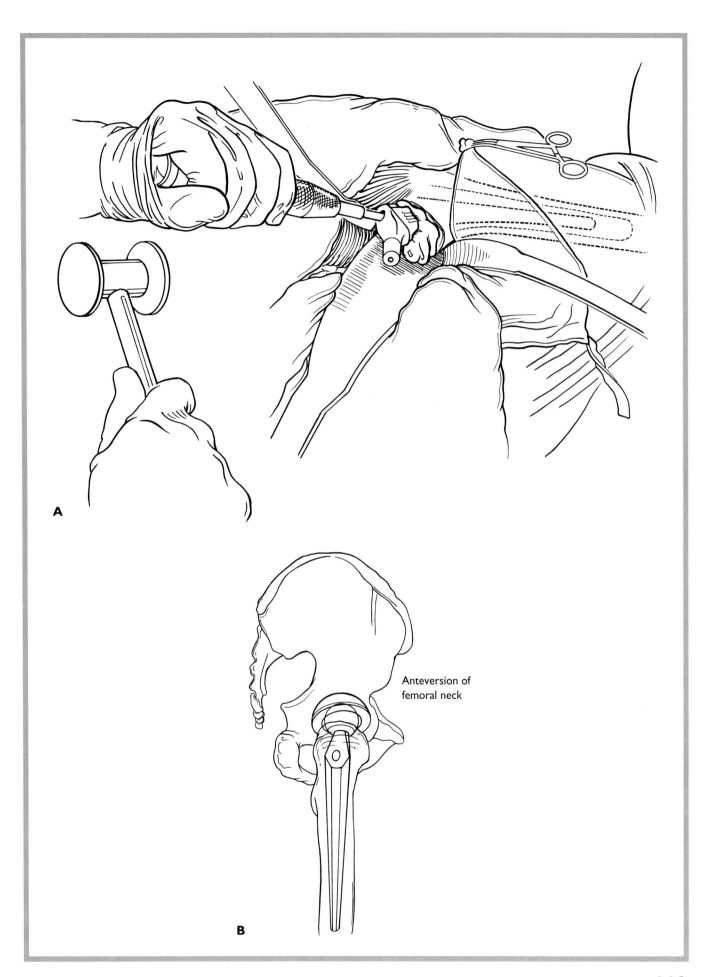

A

Anteversion of
femoral neck

B

113

Malrotation of the Femoral Component

If there is deformity of the upper femur causing retroversion or excessive anteversion to be encountered, a smaller component may be used to rotate the stem into a more neutral position. Additionally, if the cemented acetabular component has been placed in either too much or too little anteversion, a smaller femoral component can often be used to compensate by rotation in order to stabilize the hip joint.

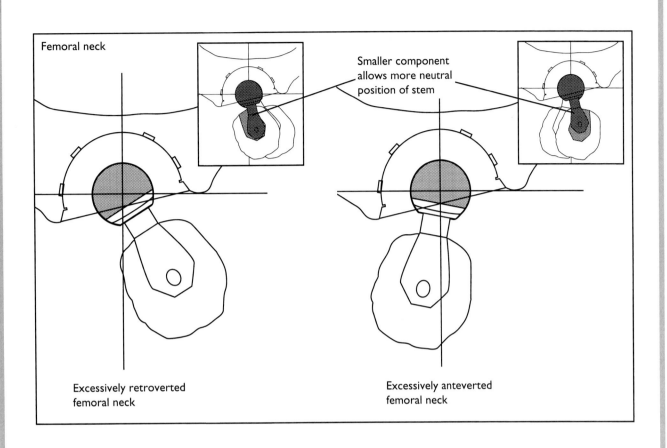

Femoral neck

Smaller component allows more neutral position of stem

Excessively retroverted
femoral neck

Excessively anteverted
femoral neck

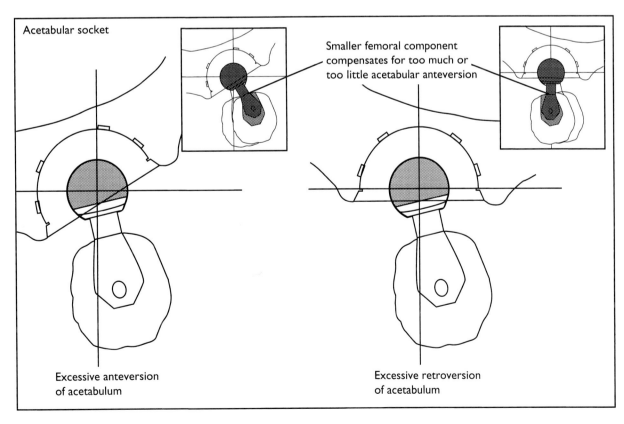

Acetabular socket

Smaller femoral component compensates for too much or too little acetabular anteversion

Excessive anteversion
of acetabulum

Excessive retroversion
of acetabulum

Femoral Component Insertion

A.

The component is held firmly until the cement has completely polymerized. In order to facilitate removal, excess cement should be
removed prior to polymerization.

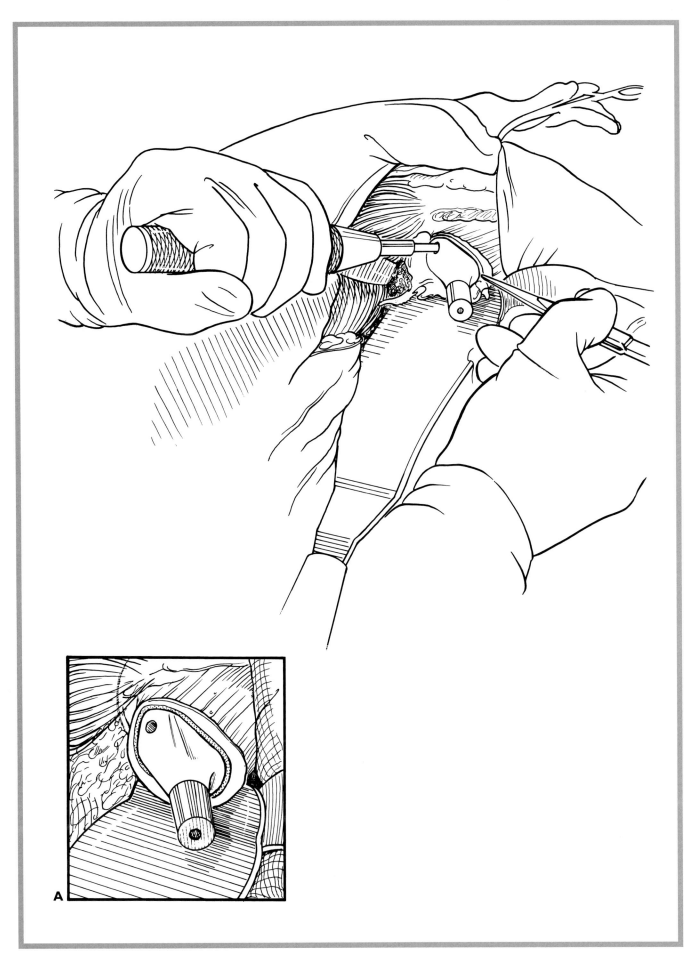

B.

Two drill holes are placed in the posterosuperior aspect of the greater trochanter.

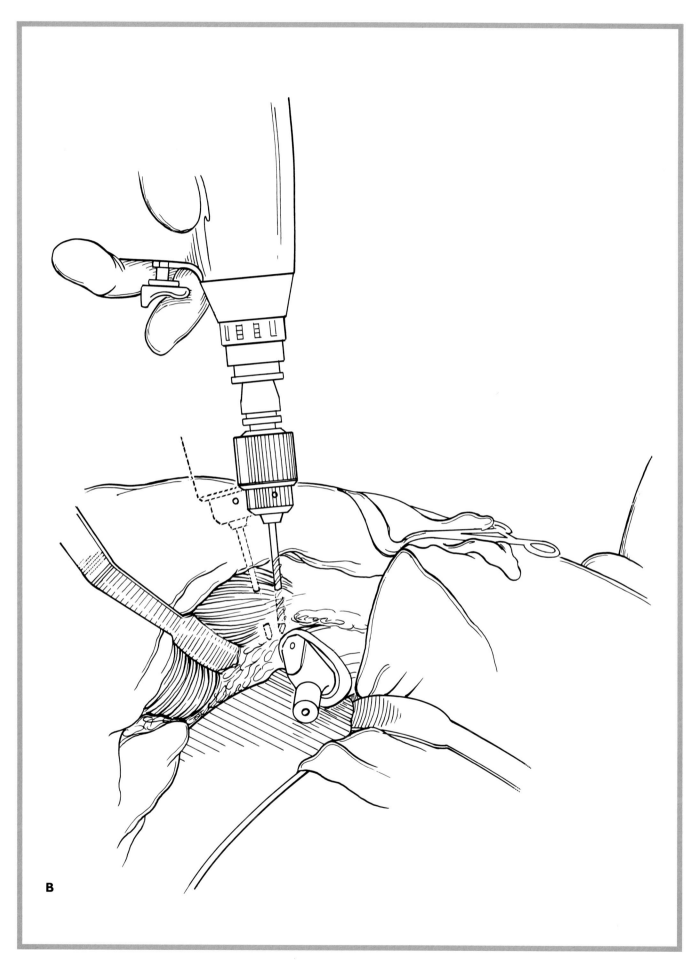

B

119

C.

Two looped sutures are passed through the drill holes for later repair of the external rotators.

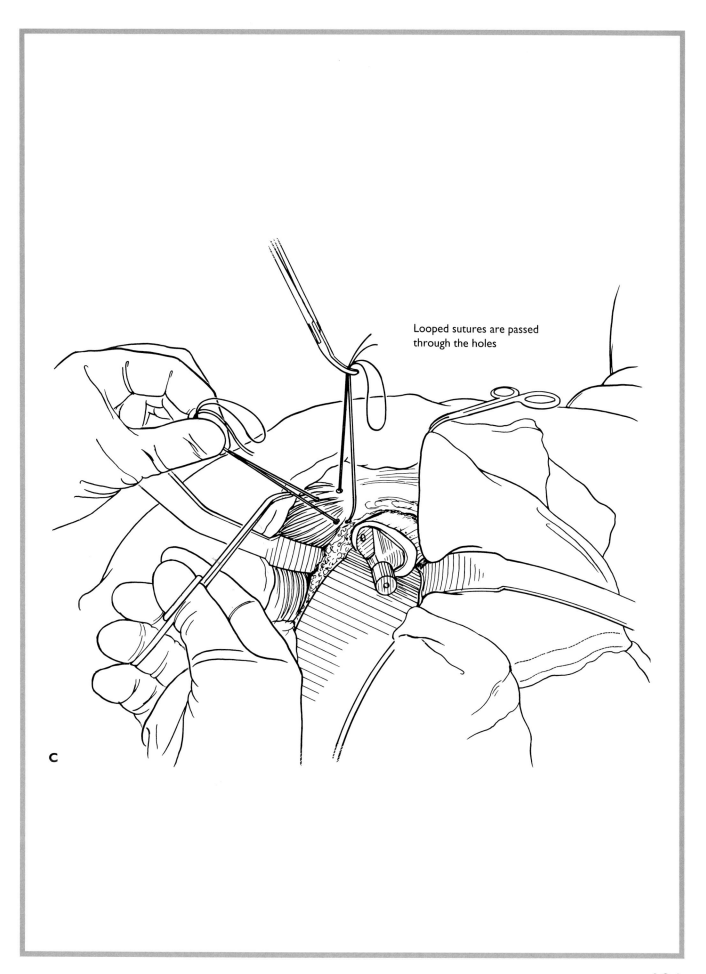

Looped sutures are passed
through the holes

c

Drain Placement

While the cement is polymerizing two suction drains are passed in a subfascial manner through the anterior thigh. A hemovac drain is attached to suction and left in place for approximately 24 hours. Drainage output over this 24-hour period is usually 300 ml. It is believed that the use of suction drains reduces the risk of wound hematoma and wound infection and may also decrease postoperative pain as the result of the reduction of joint pressure.

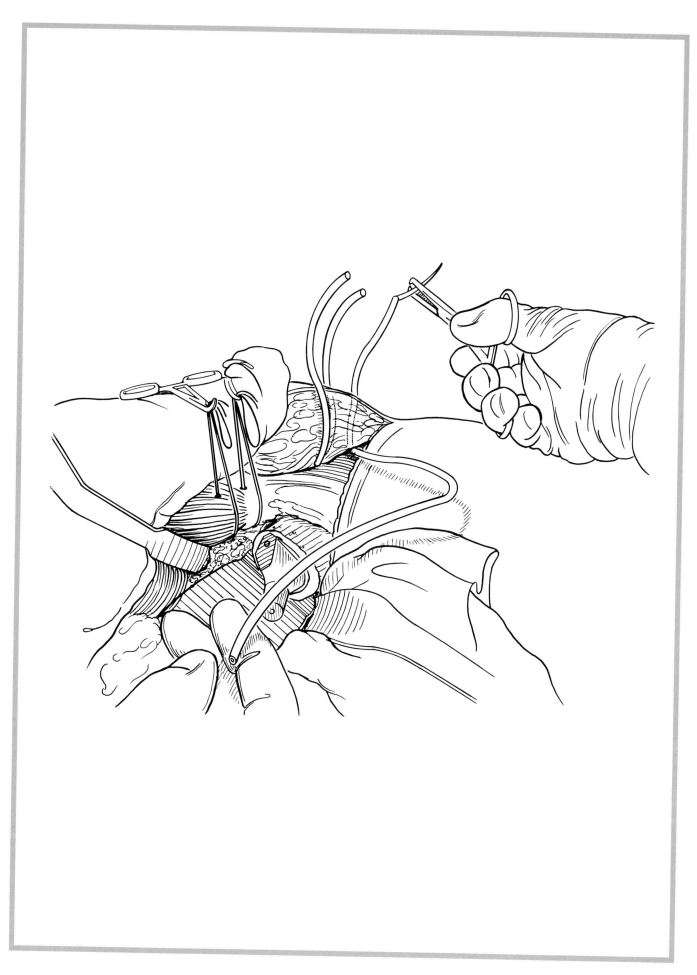

Head Replacement

A.

Care must be taken to insure that the trunion is clean and dry of cement.

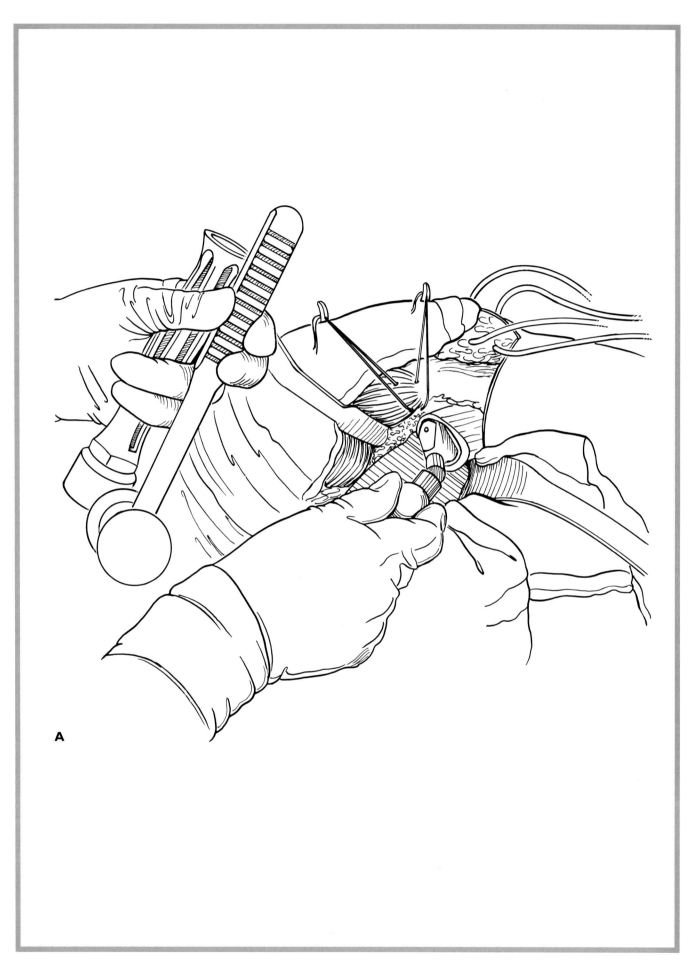

A

B.

When the cement is hardened the head is impacted gently into the trunion.

C.

An attempt is made to pull the head off to insure adequate fixation.

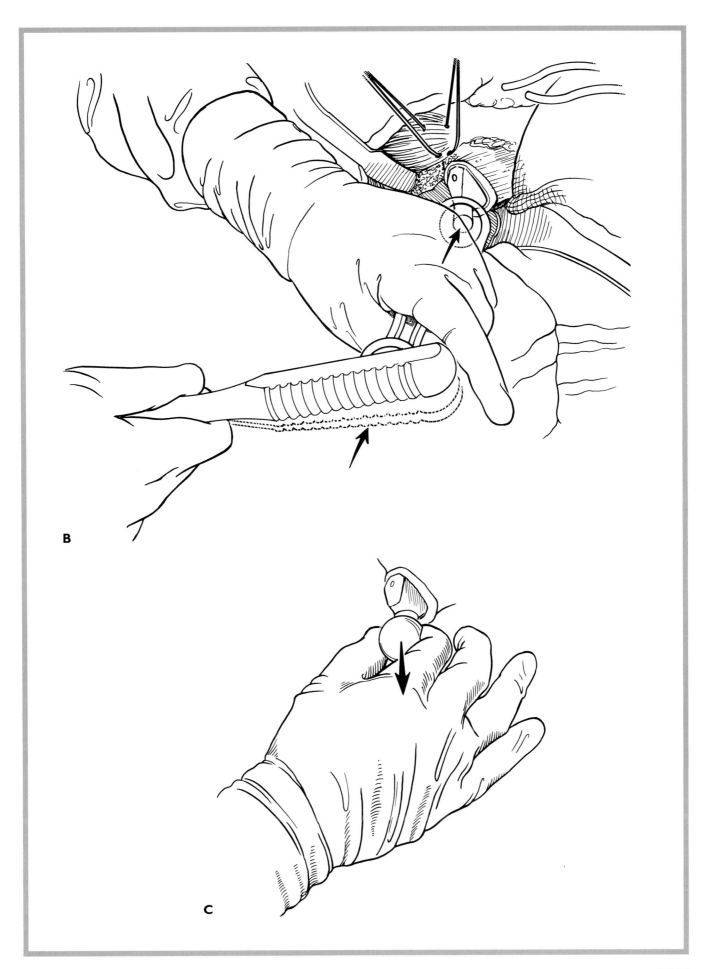

B

C

8

Hip Relocation and Closure

Relocation

A.

The hip is reduced by longitudinal traction, adduction, and internal rotation. Reassessment of hip stability is again performed. Posterior instability is assessed with flexion and internal rotation, and anterior instability is assessed with extension and external rotation.

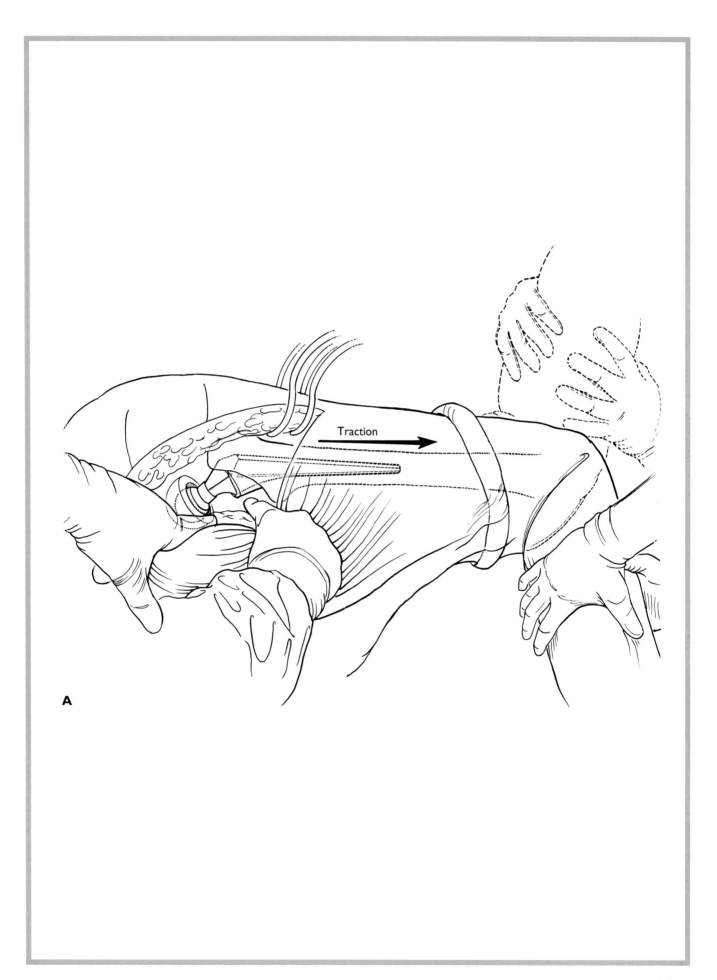

Traction

A

B.

Following assessment of stability, the leg is held in an abducted and slightly externally rotated position by resting the knee and leg on a Mayo stand.

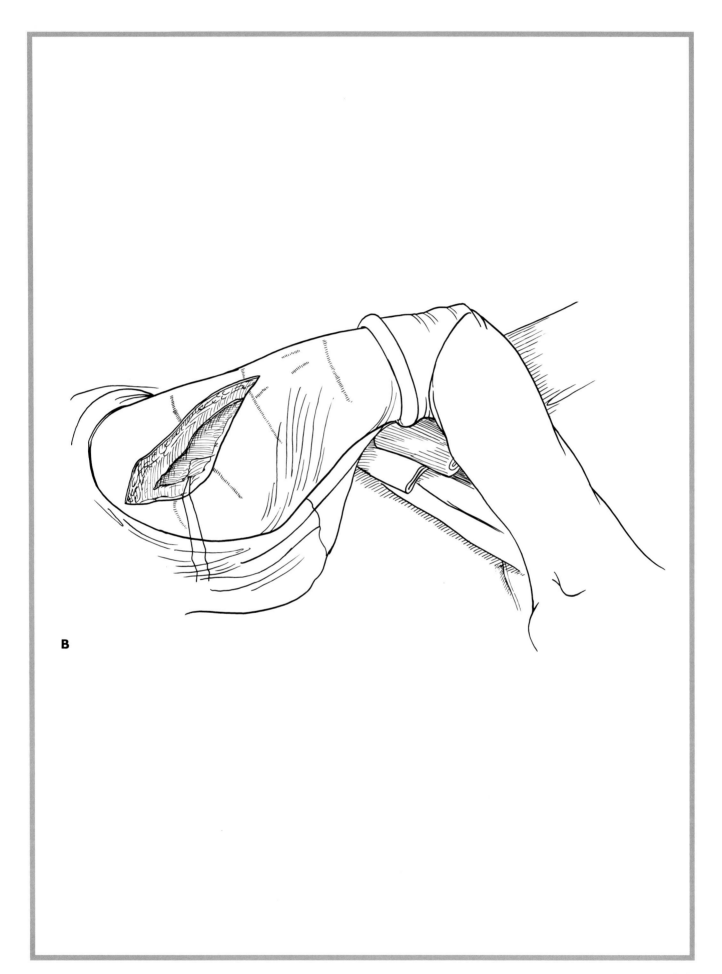

B

133

External Rotator Reattachment

The external rotators are reattached by bringing their tagging sutures through the drill holes in the greater trochanter and tying the sutures to one another over the top of the trochanter. At our institution, we decreased our dislocation rate from 4 percent to 1 percent in the late 1970s by routinely attaching the posterior structures.

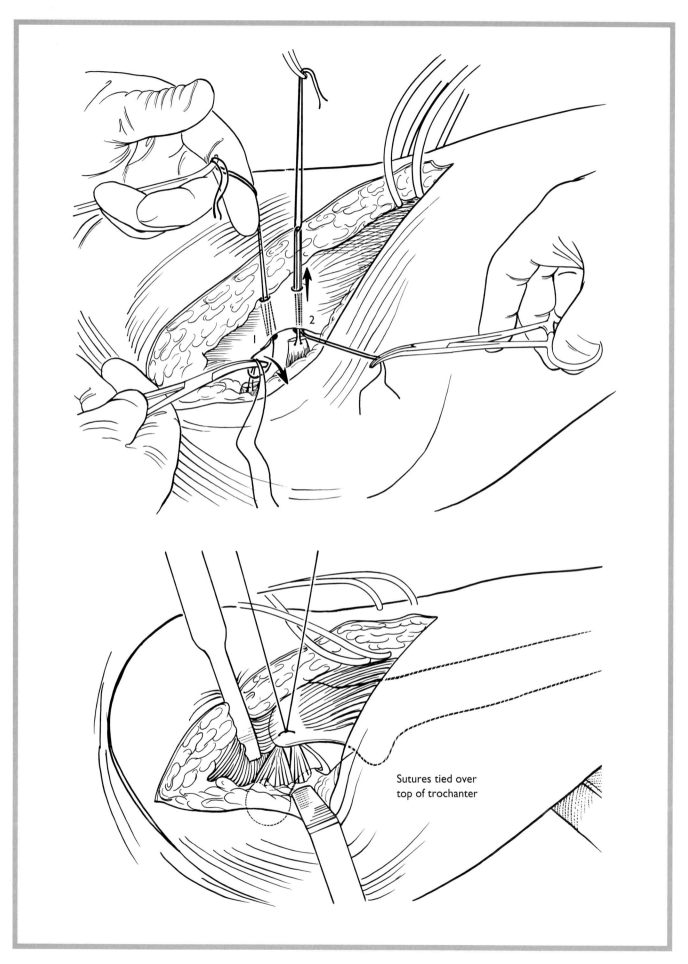

Sutures tied over
top of trochanter

135

Closure

A.

The wound is irrigated copiously with an antibiotic solution via pulsatile lavage.

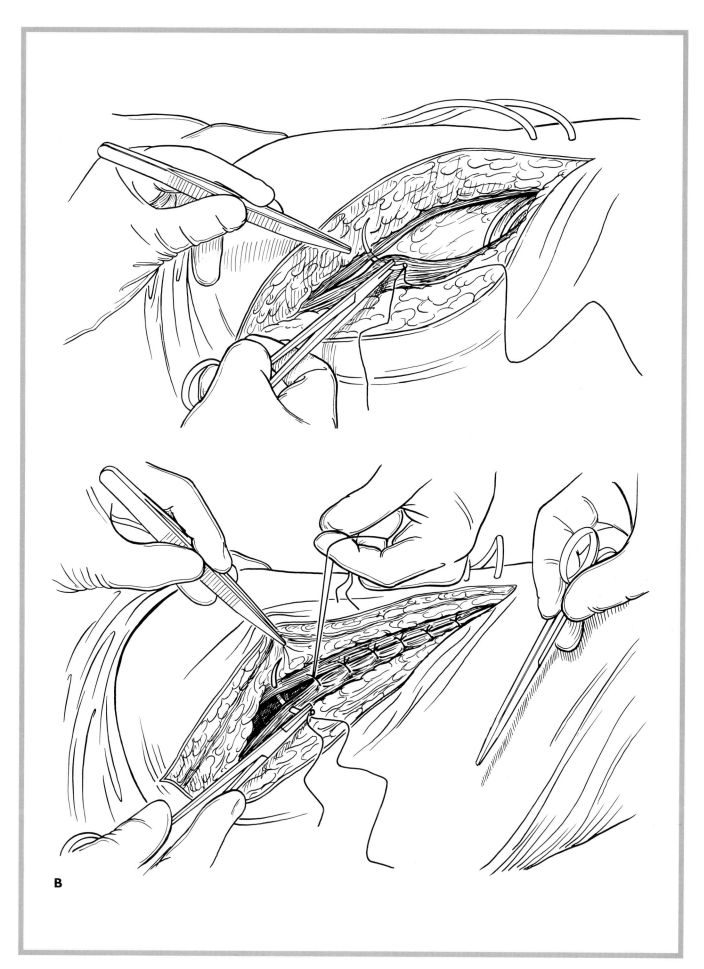

B

C.

The subcutaneous fascia is reapproximated with interrupted 2-0 vicryl
sutures.

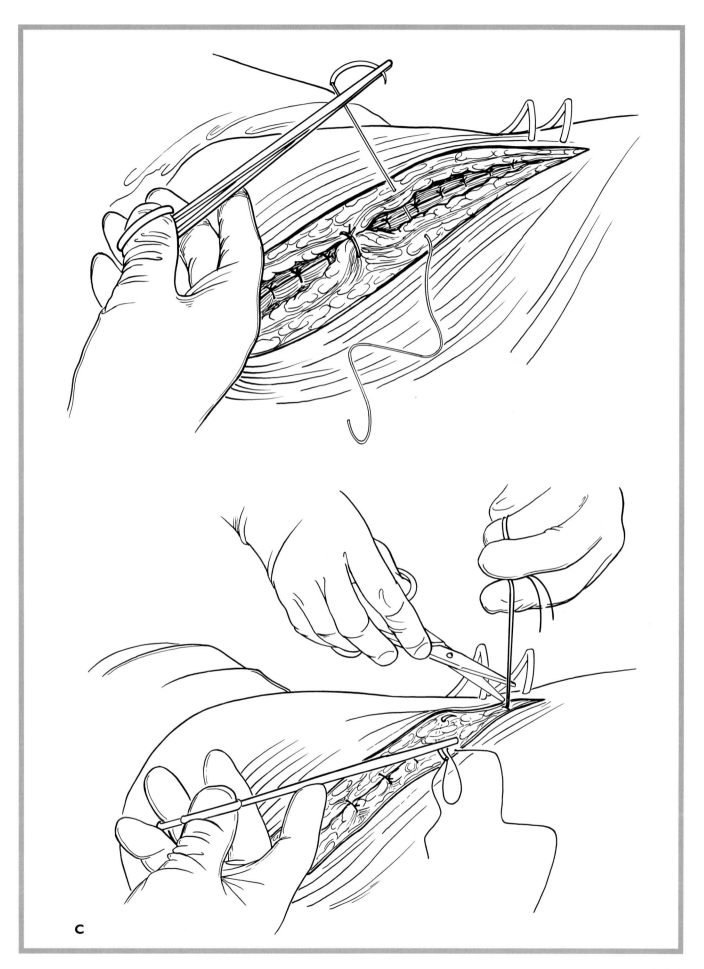

c

D.

The subcuticular layer is closed with interrupted 3-0 vicryl sutures.

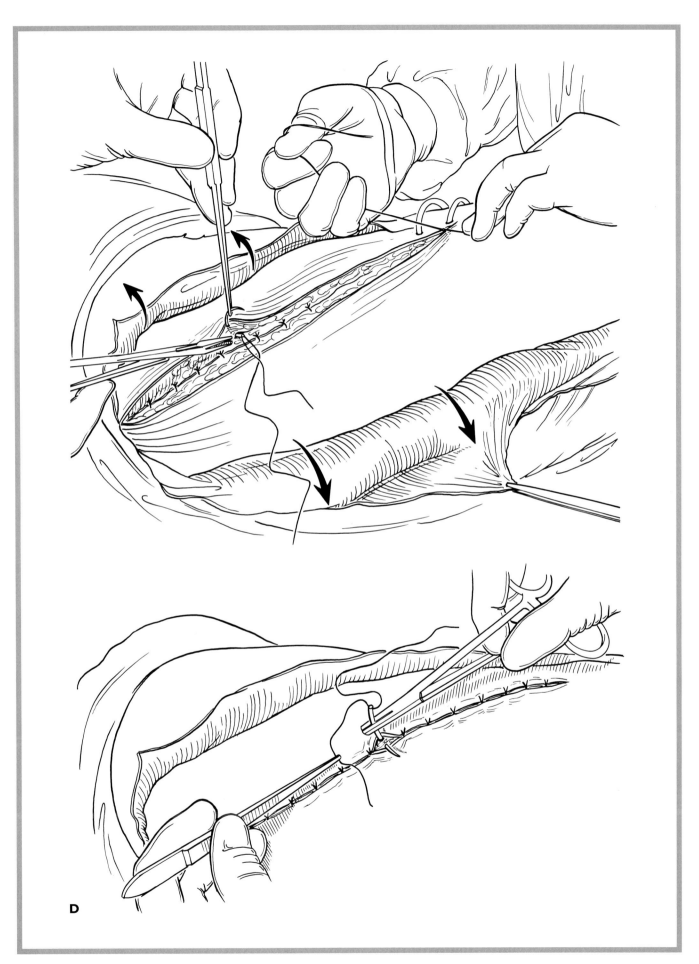

D

143

E.

The skin is closed with staples.

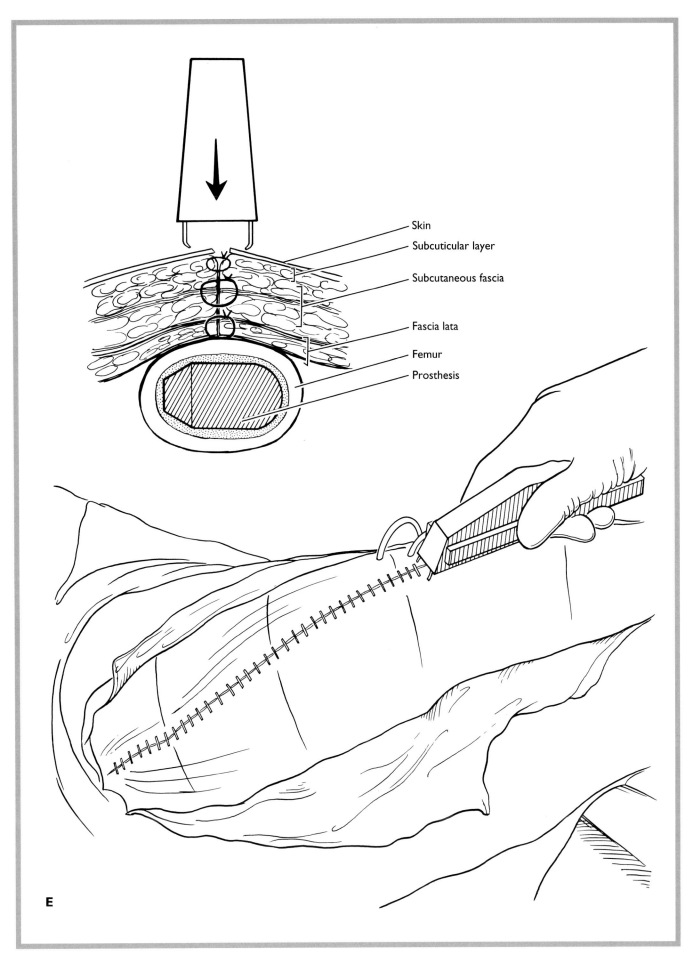

Skin

Subcuticular layer

Subcutaneous fascia

Fascia lata

Femur

Prosthesis

E

145

F.

A wet sterile dressing (4x4s) is placed over the wound. A bulky pressure dressing using an ace bandage "spica" is applied.

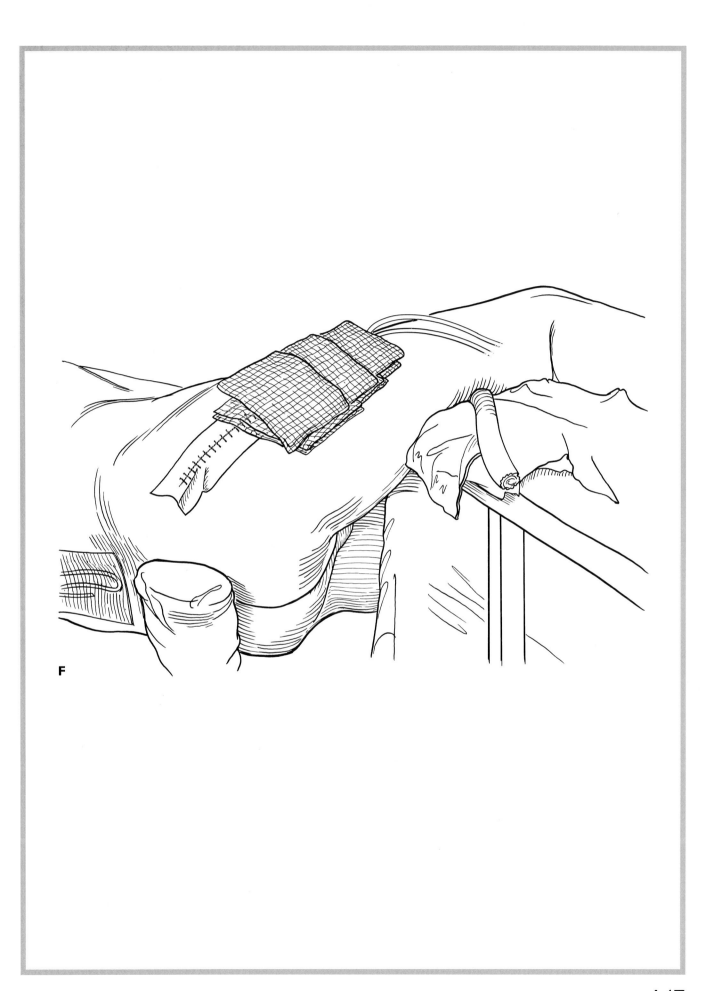

F

G.

The ace bandage is wrapped starting distally and going proximally.

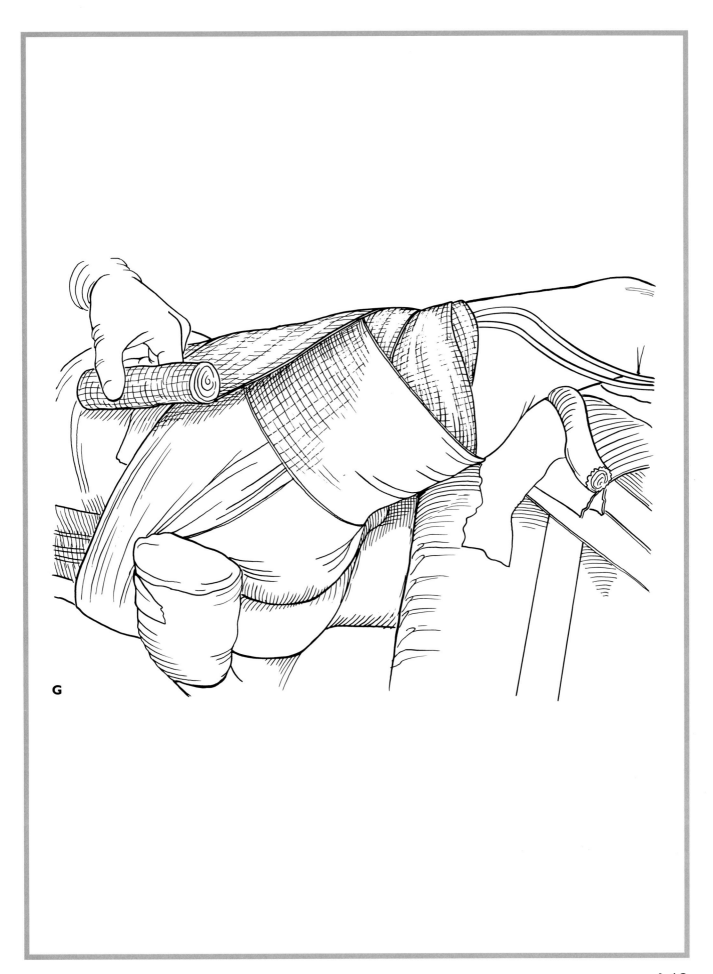

G

H.
The bandage and drains are taped to prevent removal during transport.

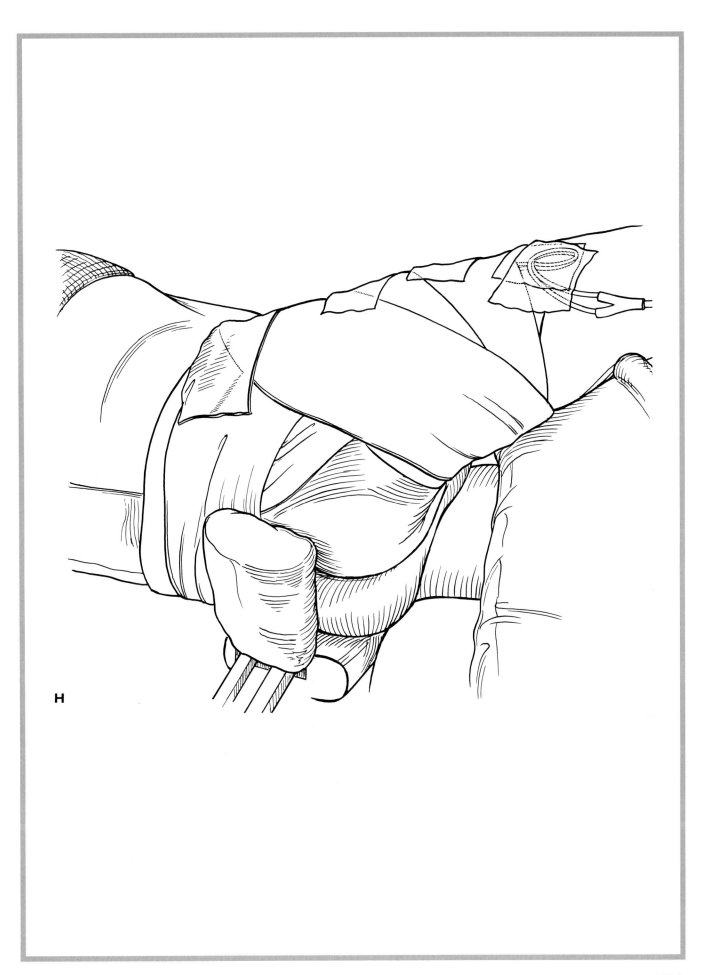

H

9

Acetabular Reaming and Sizing

Acetabular Reaming

A.

Reaming is carried out with progressively larger hemispherical grater-type reamers. The diameter of the reamers roughly match the size of the acetabular component. Reamers increase in size by 1- or 2-mm increments depending upon the system used. The use of 2-mm incremental reamers expedites acetabular preparation.

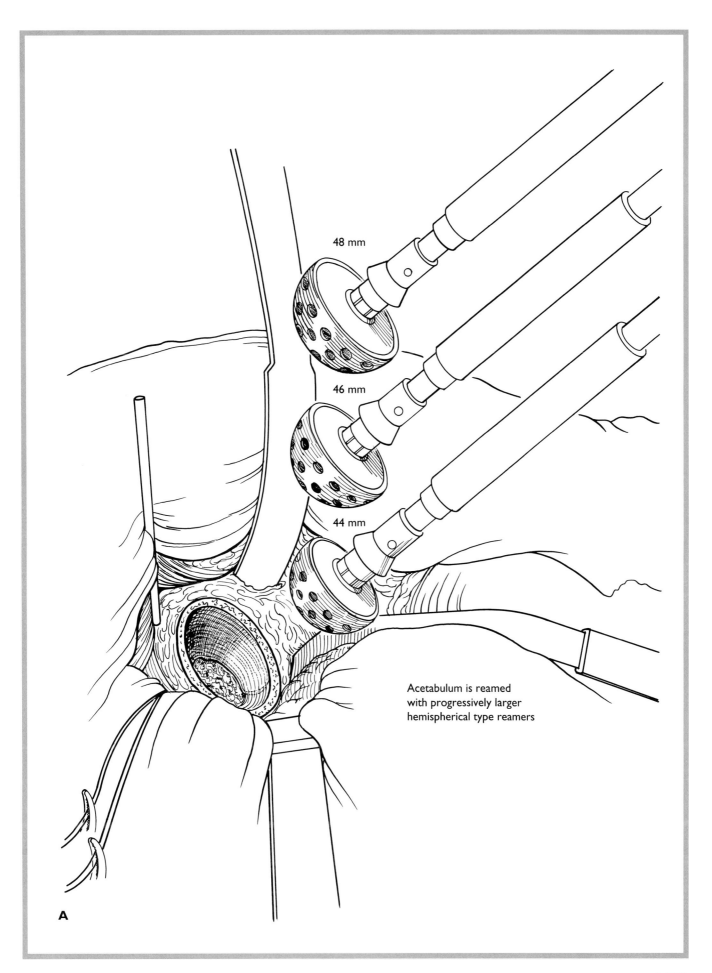

48 mm

46 mm

44 mm

Acetabulum is reamed
with progressively larger
hemispherical type reamers

A

155

B.

The pubic and ischial contributions to the acetabulum are reamed to the lateral cortex of the medial wall.

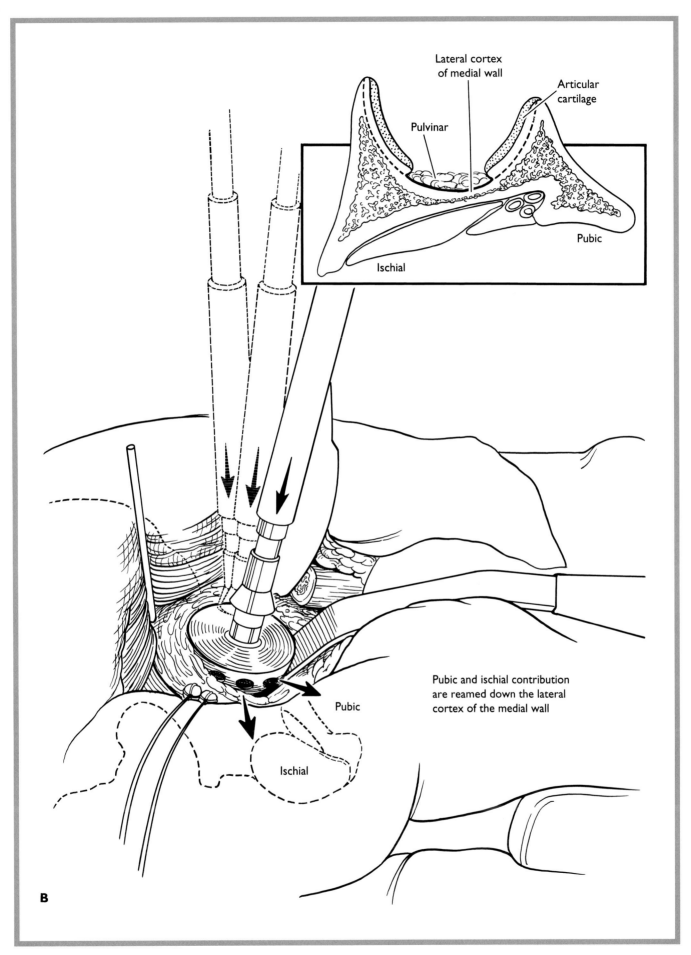

Lateral cortex
of medial wall

Articular
cartilage

Pulvinar

Ischial

Pubic

Pubic

Ischial

Pubic and ischial contribution
are reamed down the lateral
cortex of the medial wall

B

C.

The dome is reamed until the socket becomes a hemisphere. This may not be possible in cases of acetabular dysplasia. In such instances, a large enough surface of the dome should be reamed congruent with the component to provide stability.

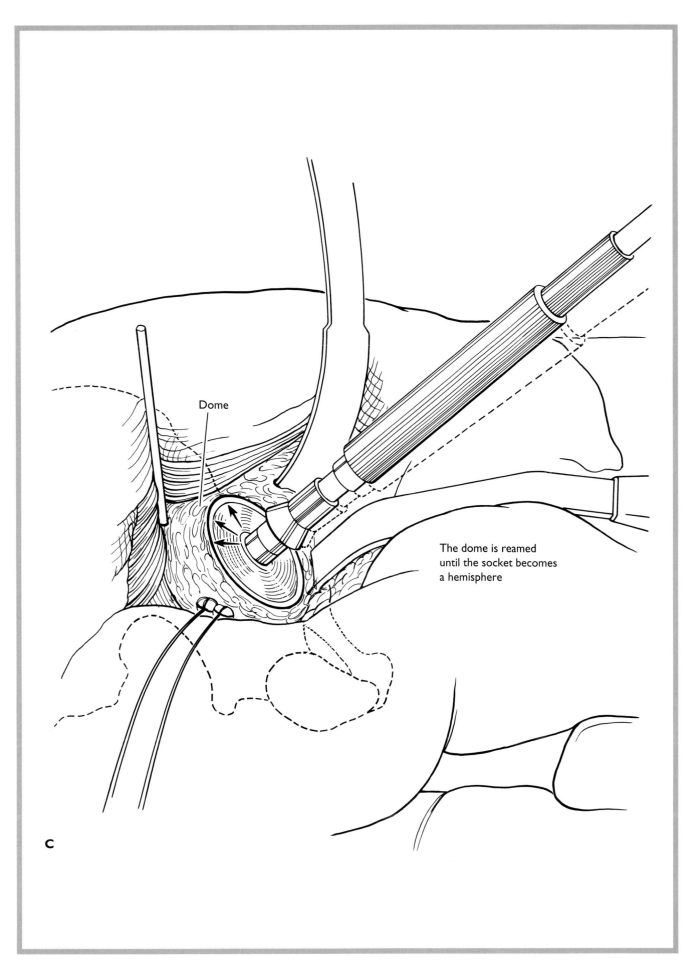

Dome

The dome is reamed
until the socket becomes
a hemisphere

c

D.

Care must be taken to avoid significant thinning of anterior and posterior walls.

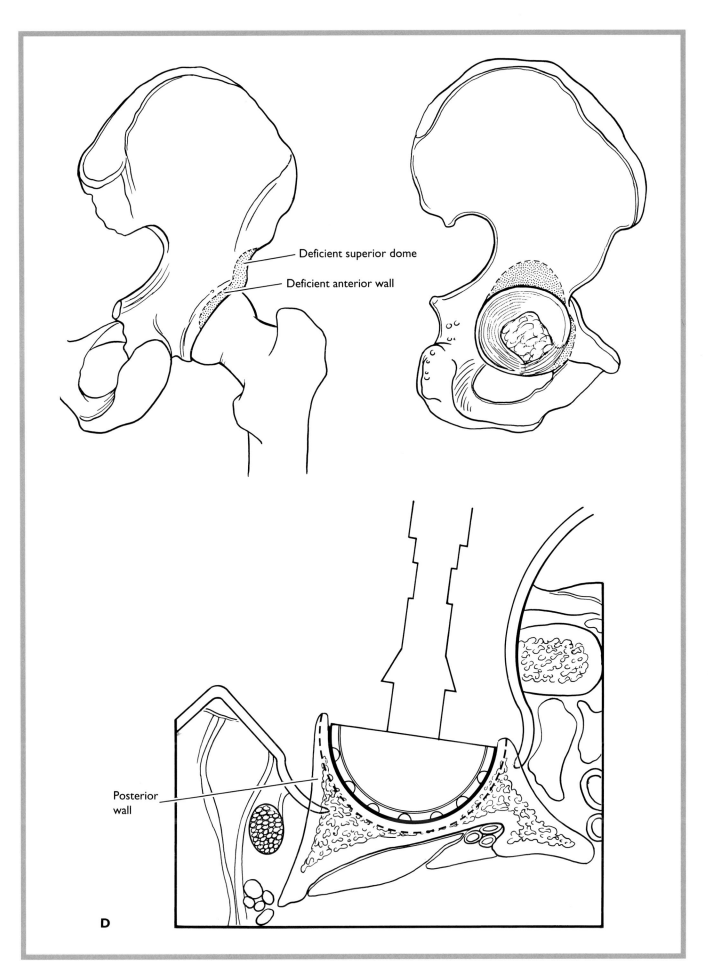

Deficient superior dome

Deficient anterior wall

Posterior
wall

D

E.

Cancellous bone should be exposed over much of the surface of the dome to provide an adequate area for potential bony ingrowth.

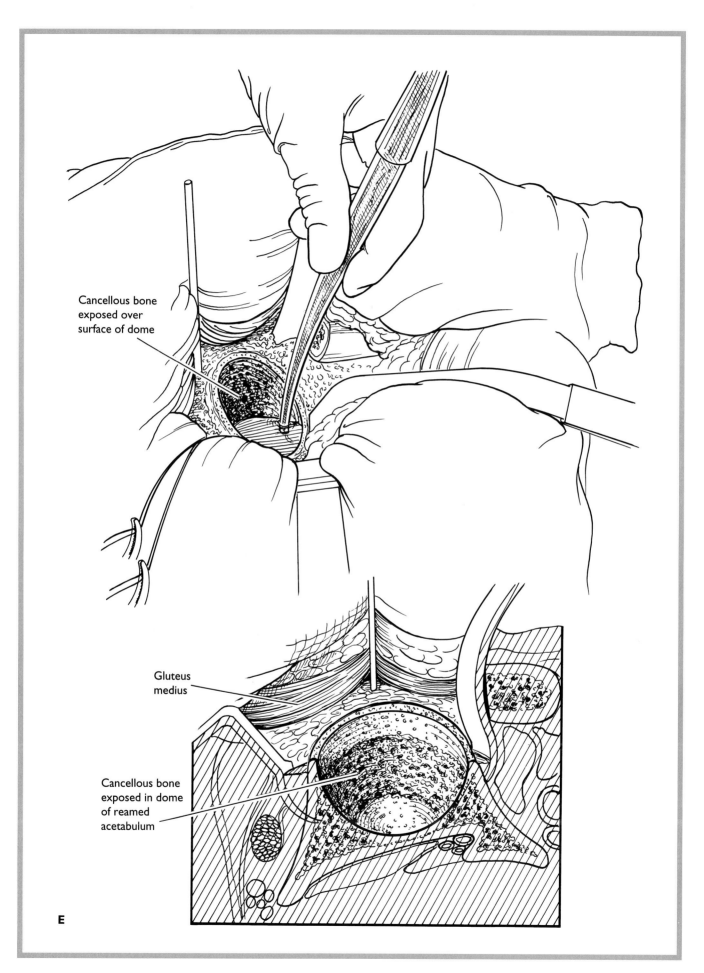

Cancellous bone
exposed over
surface of dome

Gluteus
medius

Cancellous bone
exposed in dome
of reamed
acetabulum

E

163

F.

Reaming should stop when all these parameters have been met and before the reamers become significantly uncovered (approximately 20 percent laterally).

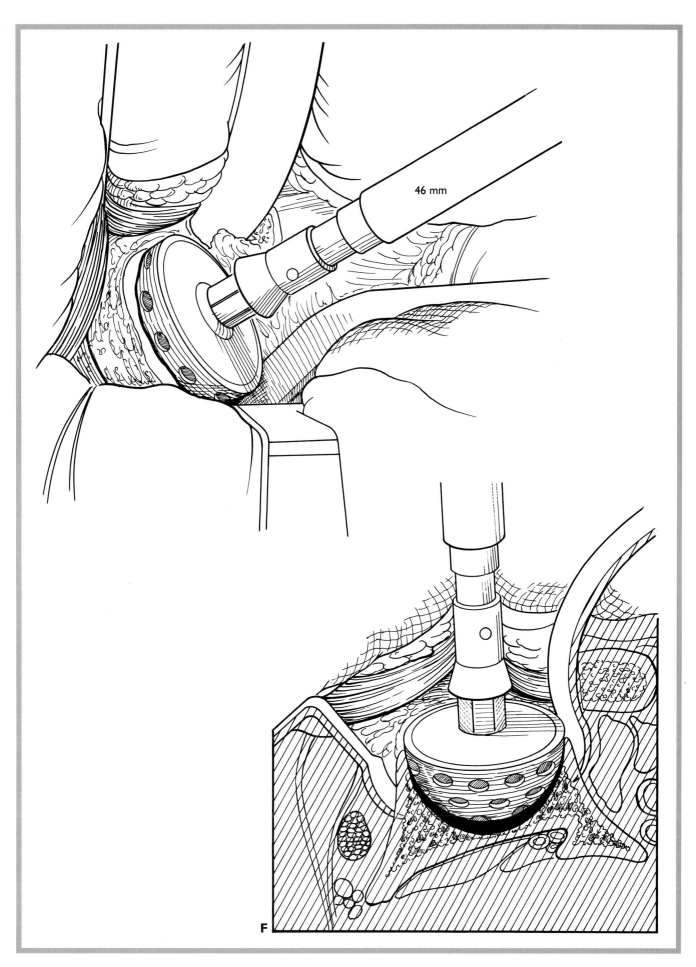

46 mm

F

Acetabular Sizing

Once bleeding cancellous bone is encountered in the ischium, pubis, and ilium, the next size reamer shell (usually 2 mm larger) can be used as a trial component. This reamer shell can give the surgeon an idea of coverage anteriorly and posteriorly, as well as in the dome. In addition, localization in the implant relative to the teardrop inferiorly is important to note at this time. The use of a 1- to 2-mm oversized implant has been advocated as a method of obtaining additional fixation during acetabular component insertion.

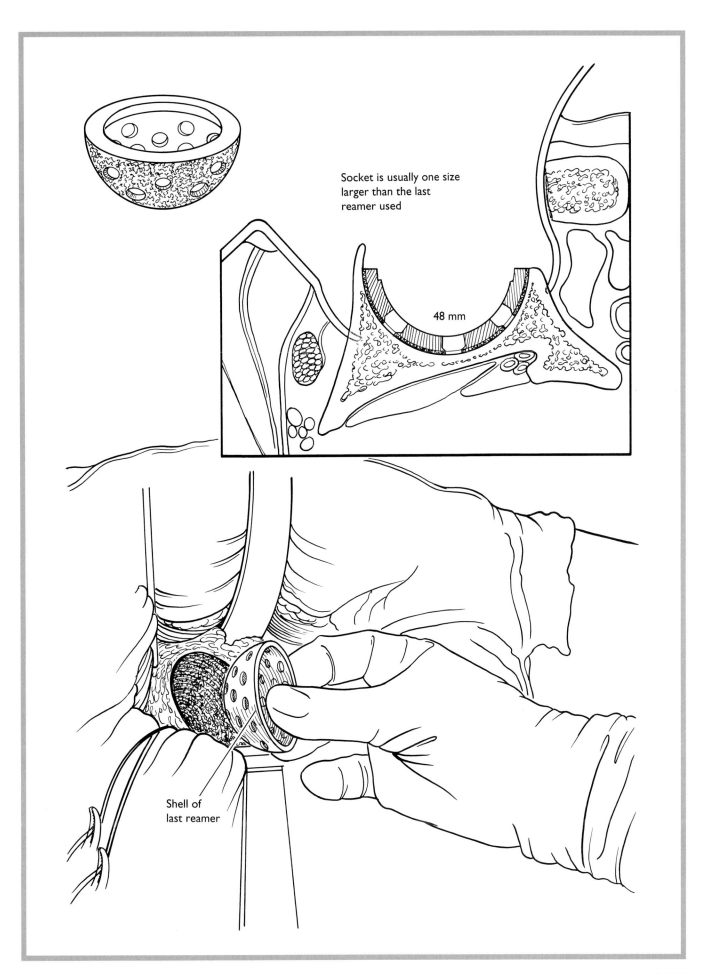

Socket is usually one size
larger than the last
reamer used

48 mm

Shell of
last reamer

167

10

Placement of Acetabular Component

Component Insertion

A.

The acetabular component is inserted with 30 to 40 degrees of abduction (inclination) and with 15 to 25 degrees of anteversion. Care must be taken to ensure that the socket is flush against the bony surfaces of the acetabulum. The socket should be kept dry. The holes in the periphery of the cup tend to fill with blood, and this makes assessment of component bone contact difficult.

B.

The acetabular insertion device should provide a firm hold on the component, yet it should release easily.

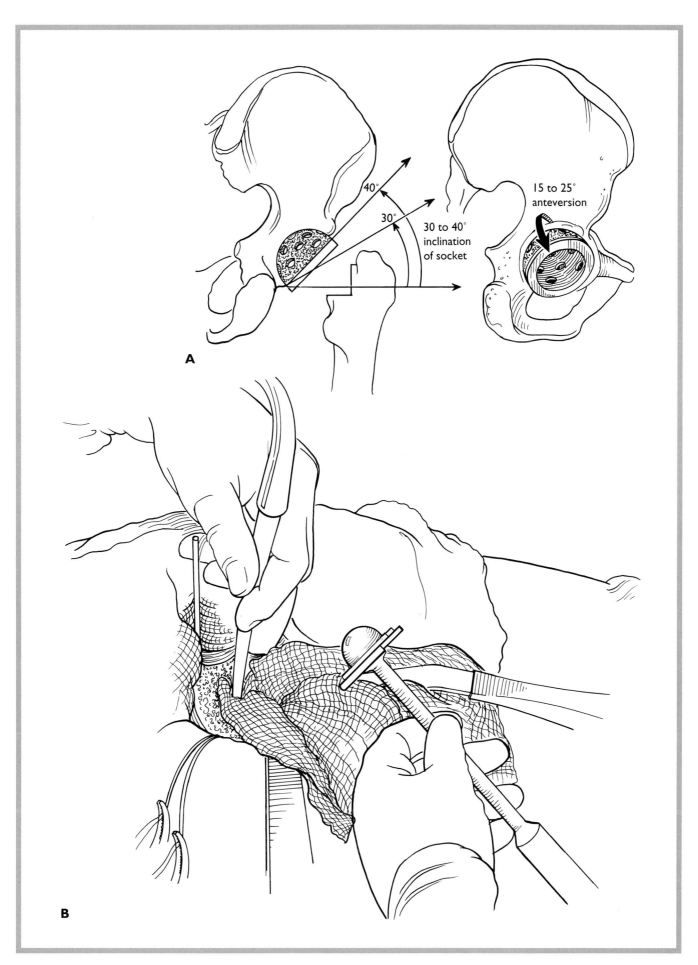

40°

30°

30 to 40°
inclination
of socket

15 to 25°
anteversion

A

B

171

C.

Using the acetabular insertion device, the component is impacted into position with a mallet. The component does not usually become flush with the underlying bony surface with this initial device. There often remains a 1- to 2-mm gap between the component and the host bone.

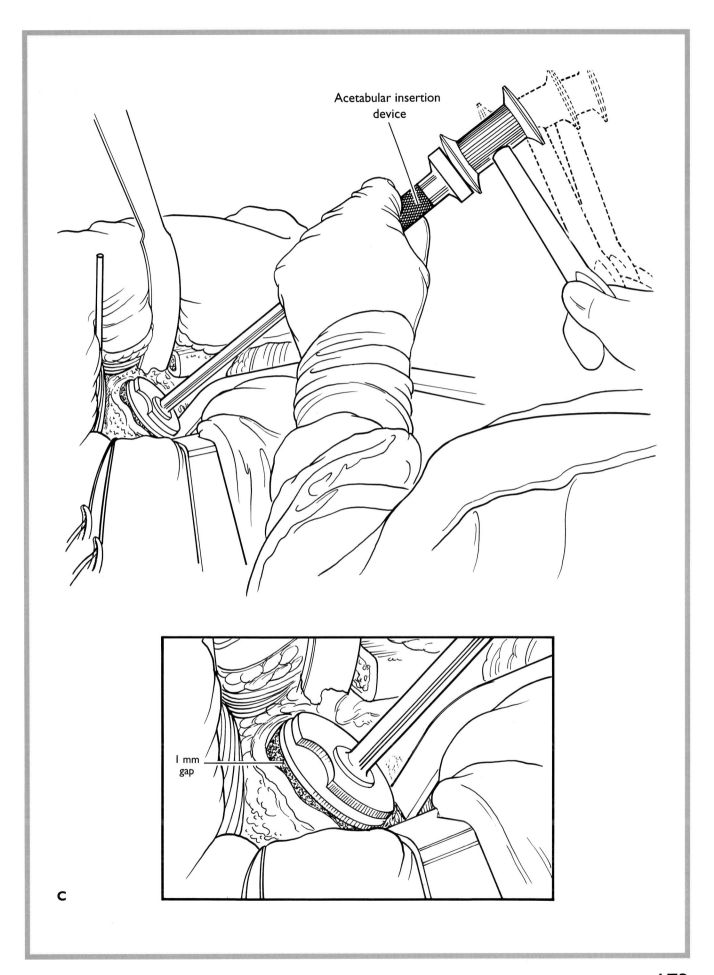

Acetabular insertion device

1 mm gap

c

D.

A ball impactor is used to "bottom out" the component to obtain implant bone contact.

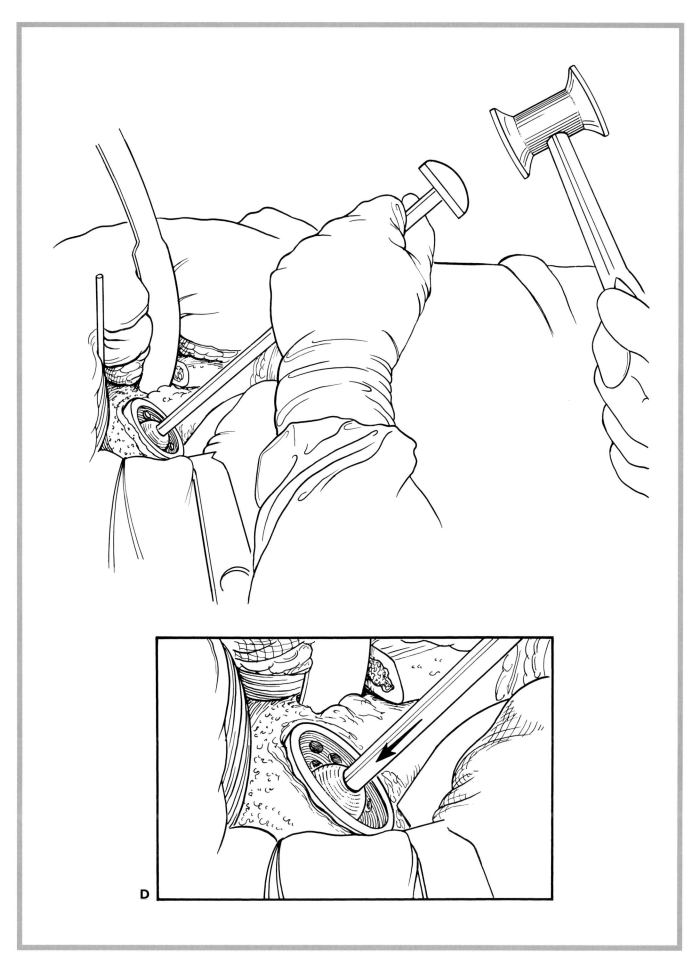

D

175

Component Fixation

A.

If component impaction leads to a tight interference fit and good implant stability, there is probably no need for the use of supplemental screw fixation. However, if there are any questions regarding fixation, one to two 6.5-mm screws are placed through the metal shell and into the wing of the ilium. The posterosuperior quadrant should be used for screw fixation to minimize the risk of penetration into the pelvis anteriorly or into the sciatic notch posteriorly. A drill guide is used to direct the medium length drill into a posterosuperior quadrant.

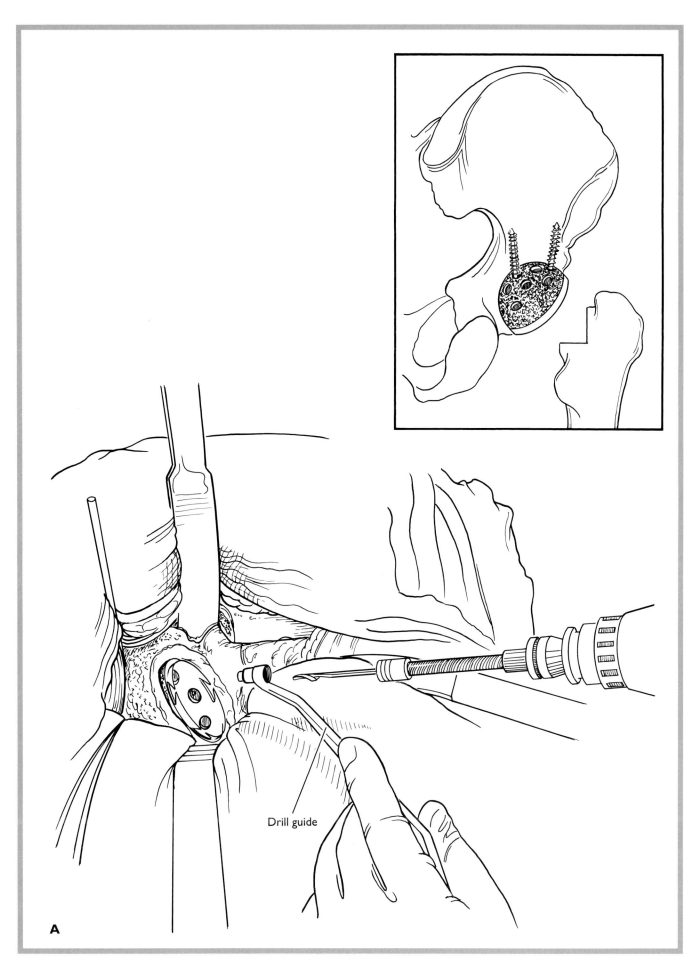

Drill guide

A

B.

The screw hole is drilled with a flexible leader on the bit to allow freedom of direction of the hole.

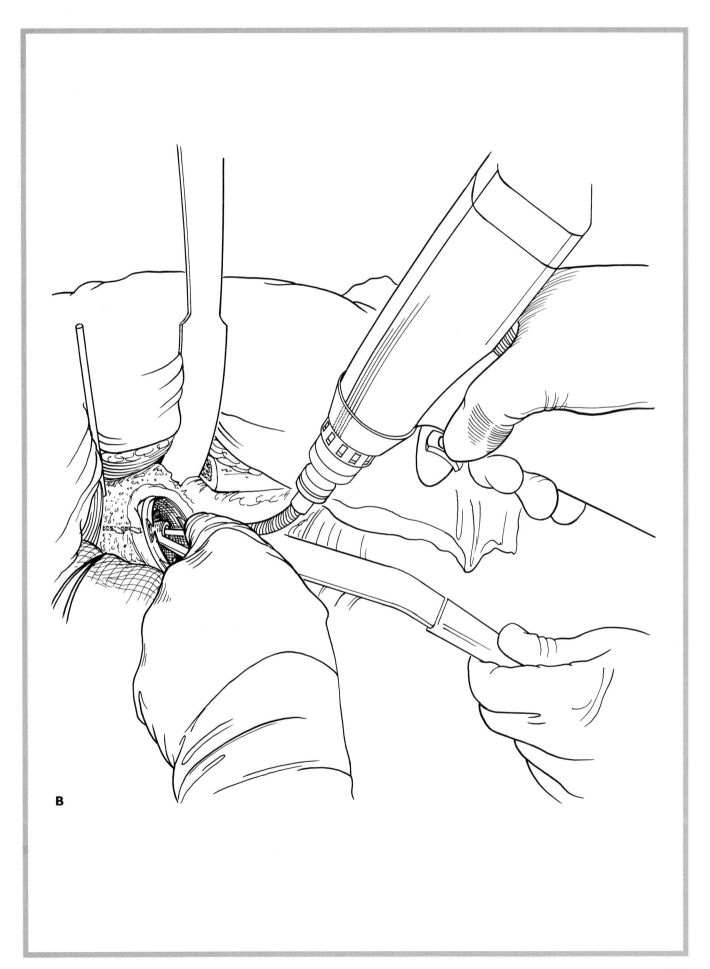

B

C.

A depth gauge is used to check the drill hole to be certain that it has not penetrated into the second cortex. The appropriate length screw is inserted (usually 20 to 30 mm). The procedure is repeated for a second screw.

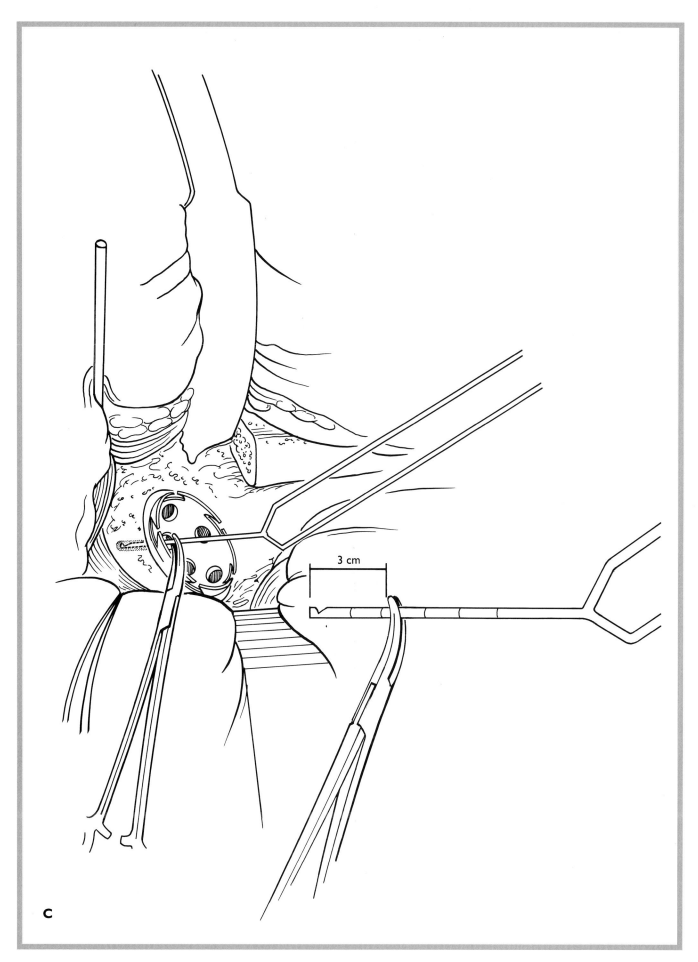

3 cm

c

D.

The wound should be lavaged freely with antibiotic solution.

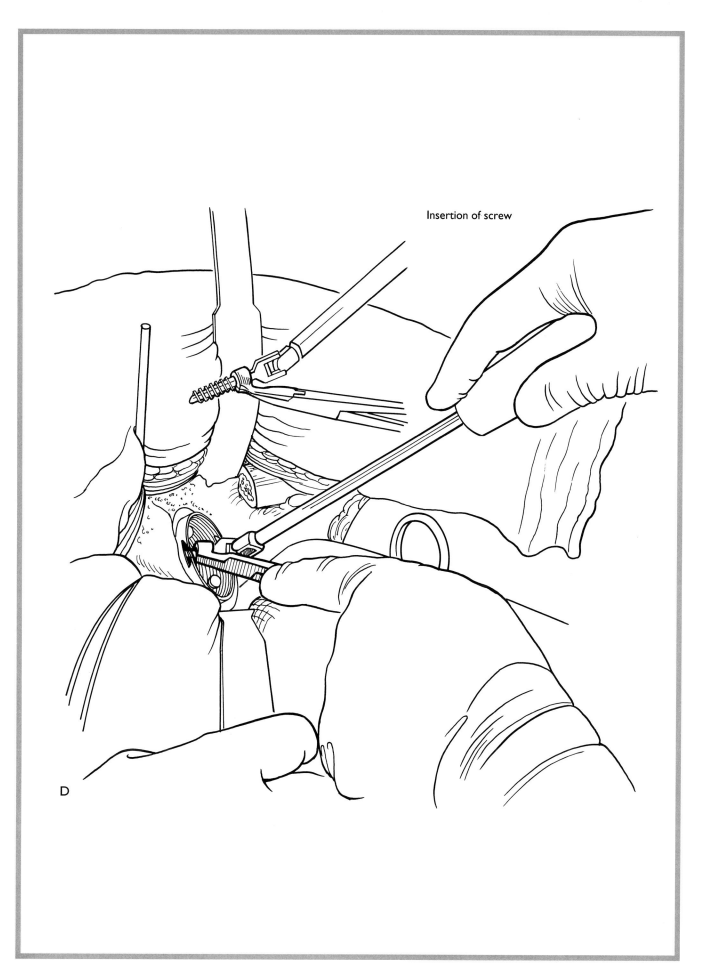

Insertion of screw

D

E.

The screw is inserted with a flexible screwdriver.

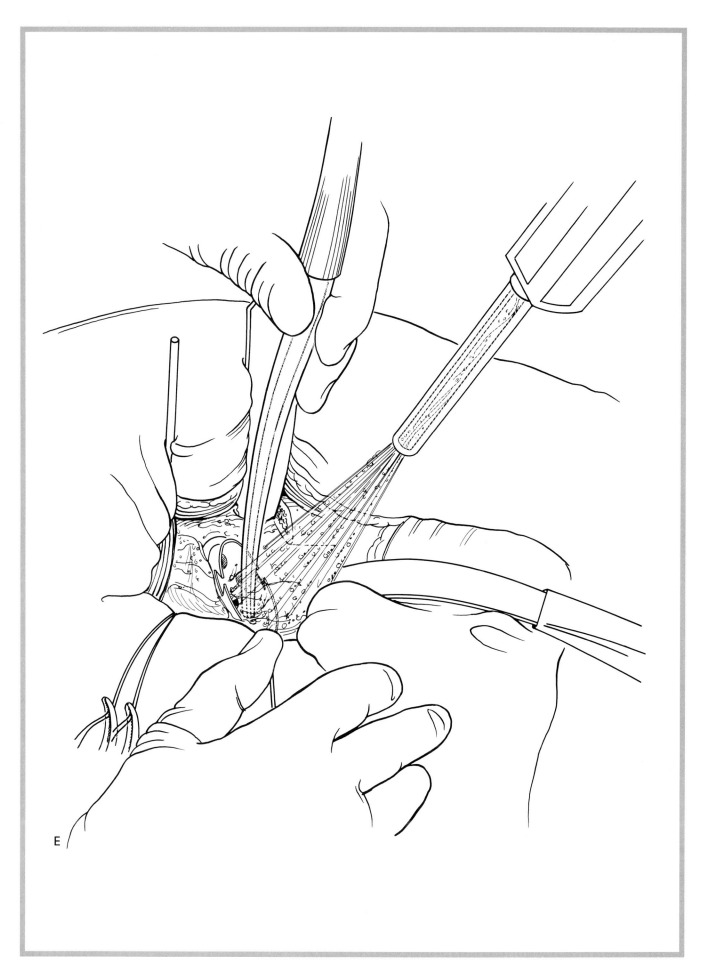

E

Insertion of Plastic Liner

A.

The locking mechanisms for the polyethylene varies greatly among manufacturers. Often, the metallic tines of the shell can be inverted slightly to improve the holding power of the polyethylene.

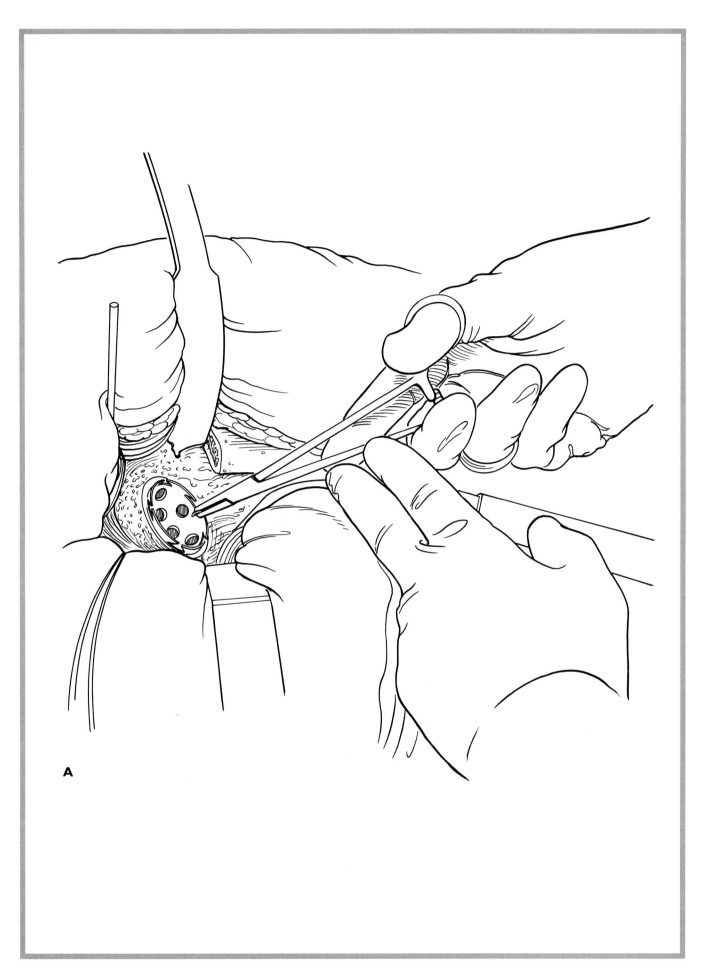

A

B.

The polyethylene insert is now placed into the acetabular component opening. The use of flat or elevated liner rims is usually a matter of surgeons' preference but may afford added stability to the hip.

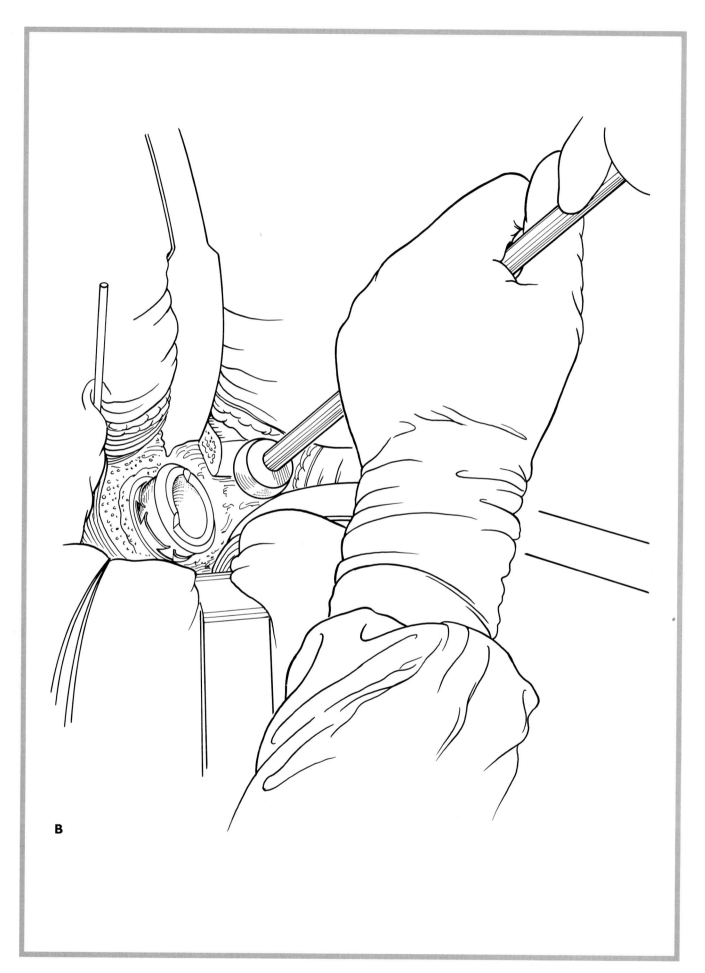

B

C.

The plastic liner is impacted until it seats within the metal shell. At this point the anesthesiologist gives the patient 1,000 mg of heparin. A study performed a few years ago demonstrated that heparin reduces the postoperative incidence of thromboembolic disease. The length of time of the surgery is also related to the incidence of blood clots in the thigh and leg. The most likely cause of the clots is the twisting of the femoral vein when the femur is exposed. Administration of heparin just before the femoral side is done ensures that the leg is full of heparin when it is twisted.

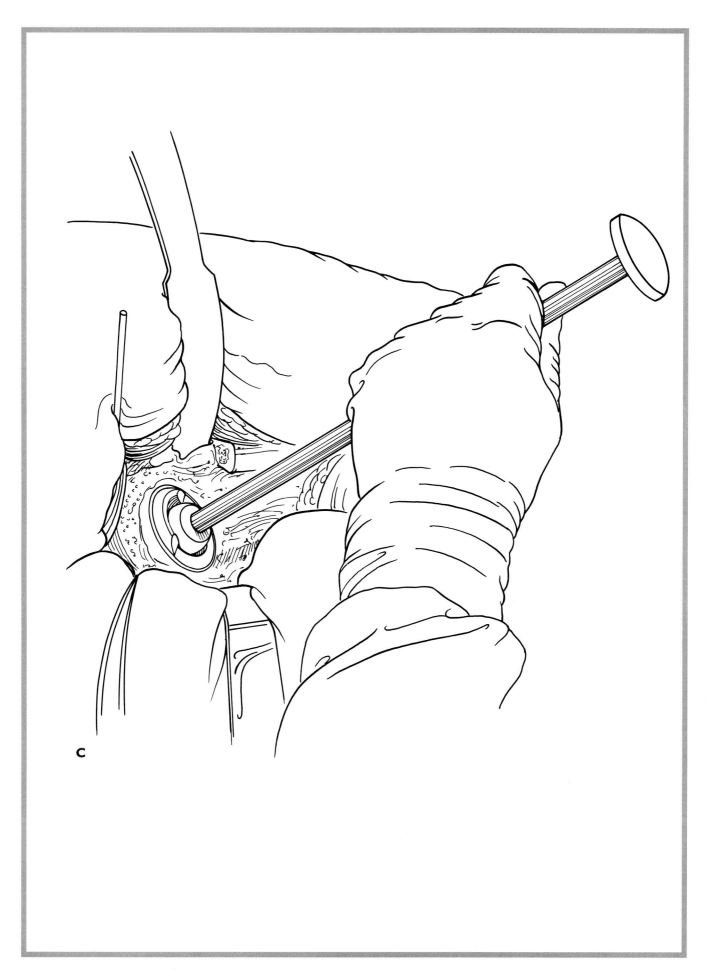

c

11

Femoral Reaming and Broach Trials

Cementless Femoral Reaming

A.

Reaming of the canal is initiated with cylindrical reamers.

B.

The neck should be entered laterally directly overlying the femoral canal to avoid varus or valgus reaming.

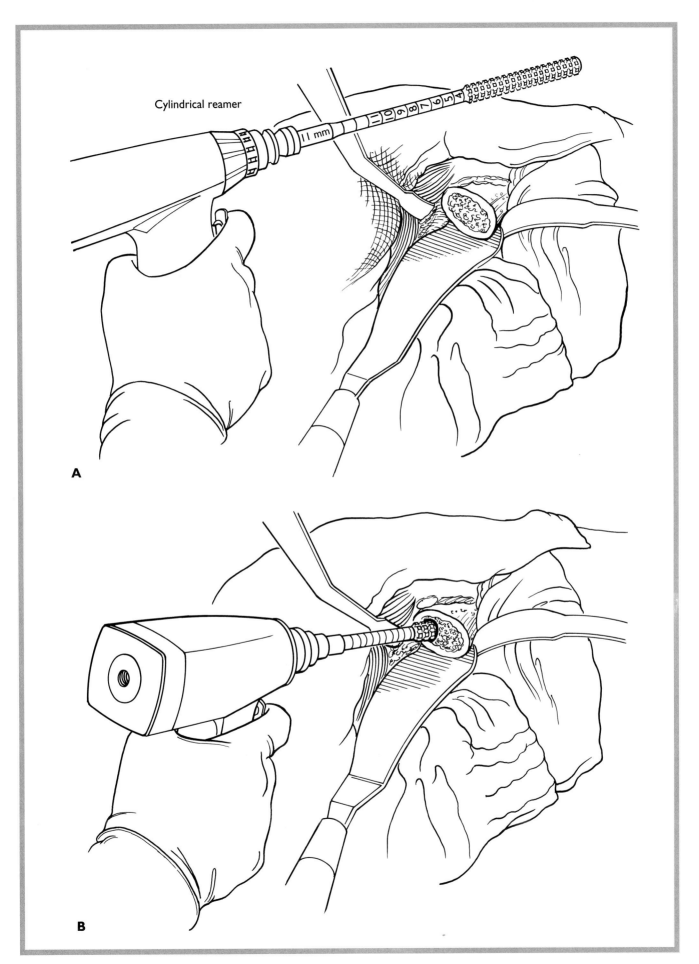

Cylindrical reamer

A

B

C.

Femoral templates are used preoperatively to determine the size of the prosthesis that will optimize hip biomechanics and restore limb length. Care should be used to correctly orient the templates in relation to the lesser trochanter. Reamers are marked accordingly and inserted to appropriate length.

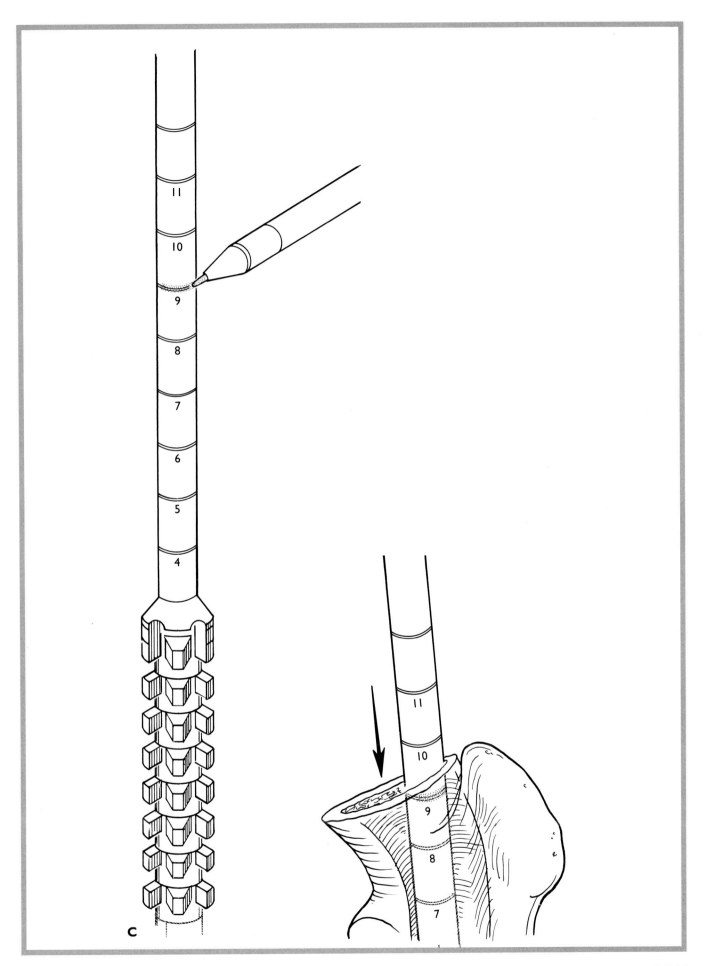

D.

Progressively larger diameter cylindrical reamers (1-mm increments) are used until endosteal cortex is encountered. Depending upon the resistance encountered, reaming should be discountinued at this diameter or continued to one size larger. The diameter of the reame should correspond to the diameter of the modular distal tip, measured preoperatively using femoral templates, within 1 mm.

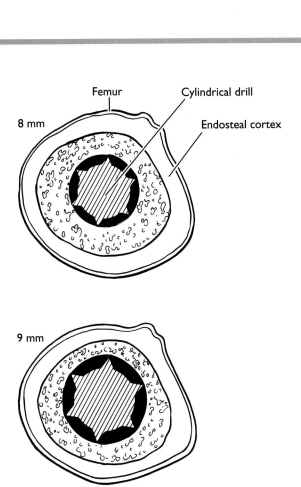

8 mm — Femur — Cylindrical drill — Endosteal cortex

9 mm

10 mm

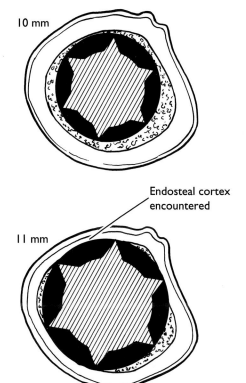

Endosteal cortex
encountered

11 mm

D

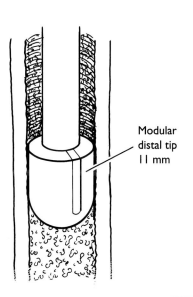

Modular
distal tip
11 mm

E.

The adequacy of reaming should be tested with a trial tip insertion device.

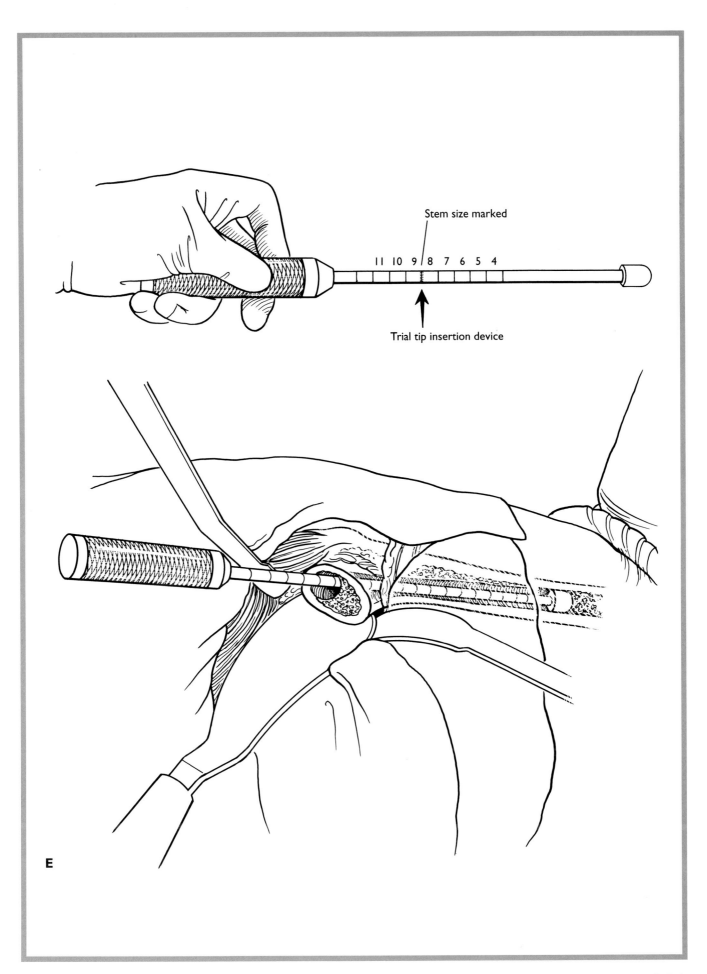

Stem size marked

11 10 9 8 7 6 5 4

Trial tip insertion device

E

Broach Trials

A.

Reaming is continued with broaches. It is recommended to begin with one to two sizes below the final anticipated size.

B.

The proper diameter tip should be *firmly* affixed to the broach device trial.

C.

Broaching is performed with gentle repetitive tapping blows to the insertion handle. Care should be taken to ensure proper orientation of the broach handle. It is imperative that the broach not be inserted in a varus orientation. Varus insertion of the broach almost certainly leads to undersizing of the implant. When the broach stops advancing, impaction should be discontinued or femur fracture may occur.

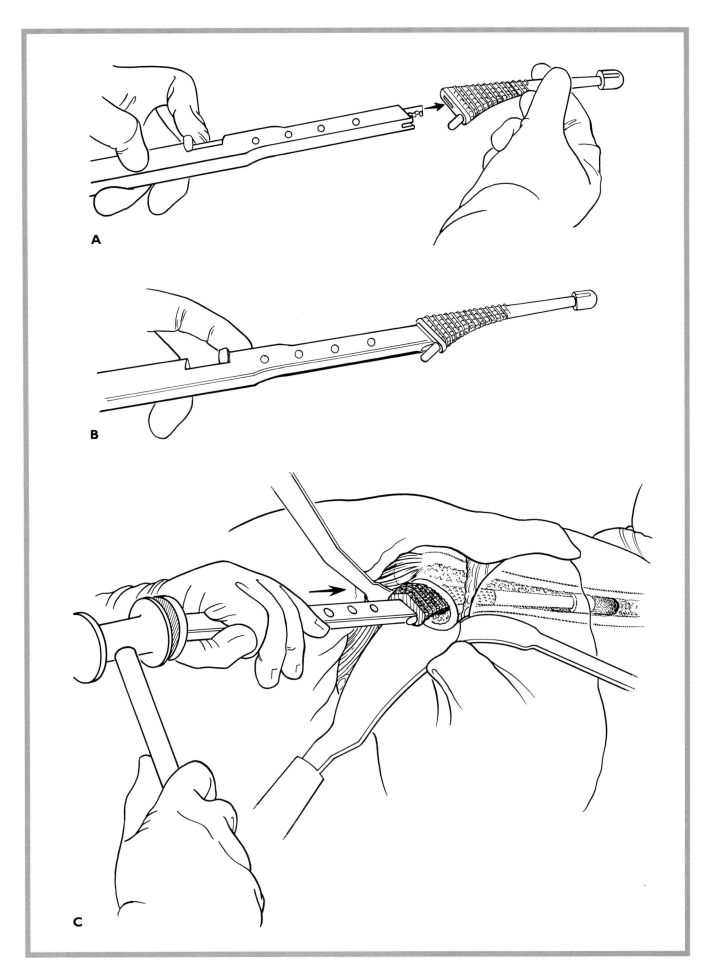

D.

The broach is removed and the reamed cross-section of the femoral neck should be assessed in relation to the size of the broach.

E.

If there is more than 1 to 2 mm of cancellous bone remaining on the posterior endosteal surface, it is usually possible to advance to the next broach size.

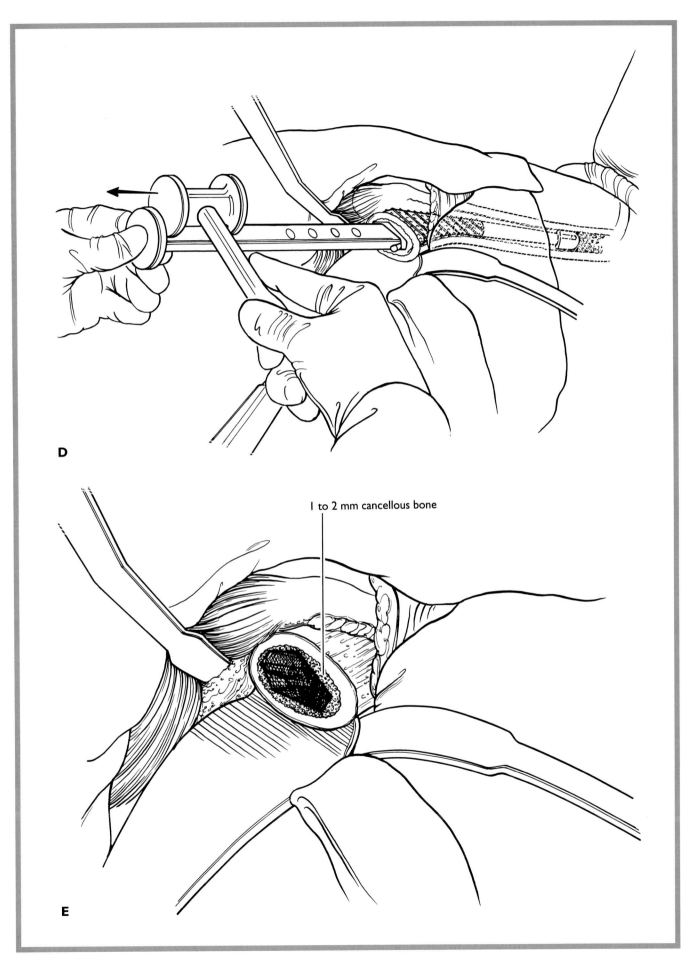

D

1 to 2 mm cancellous bone

E

F.

With the final-sized trial broach in place, the insertion handle is removed and the provisional neck/head assembly is attached to the broach.

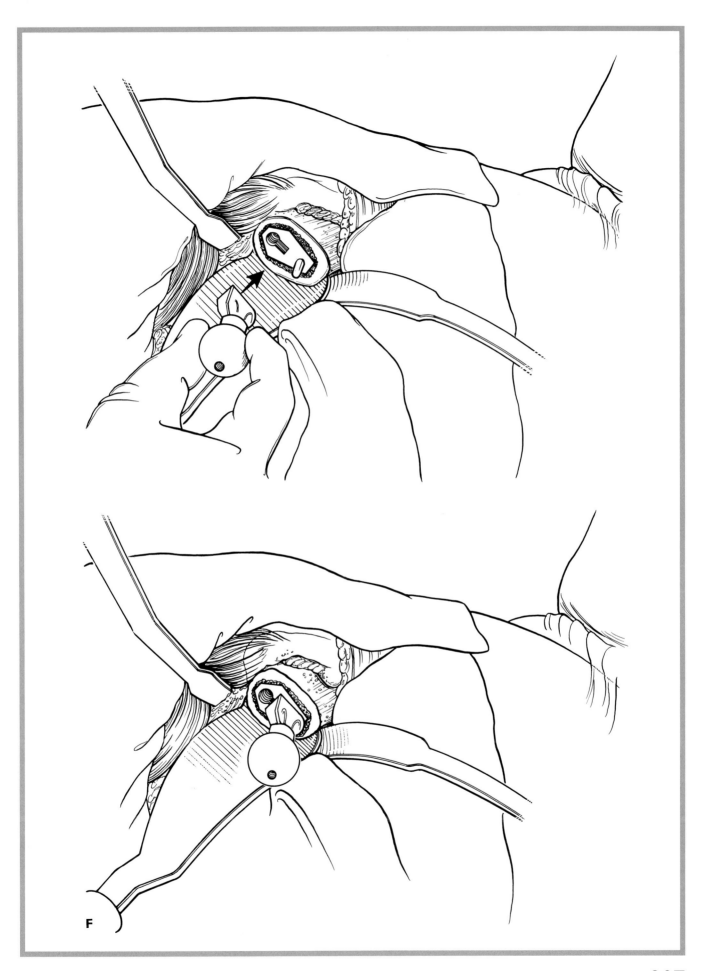

G.

The lesser trochanter to center of femoral head distance should match that measured for the contralateral hip during preoperative template measurements.

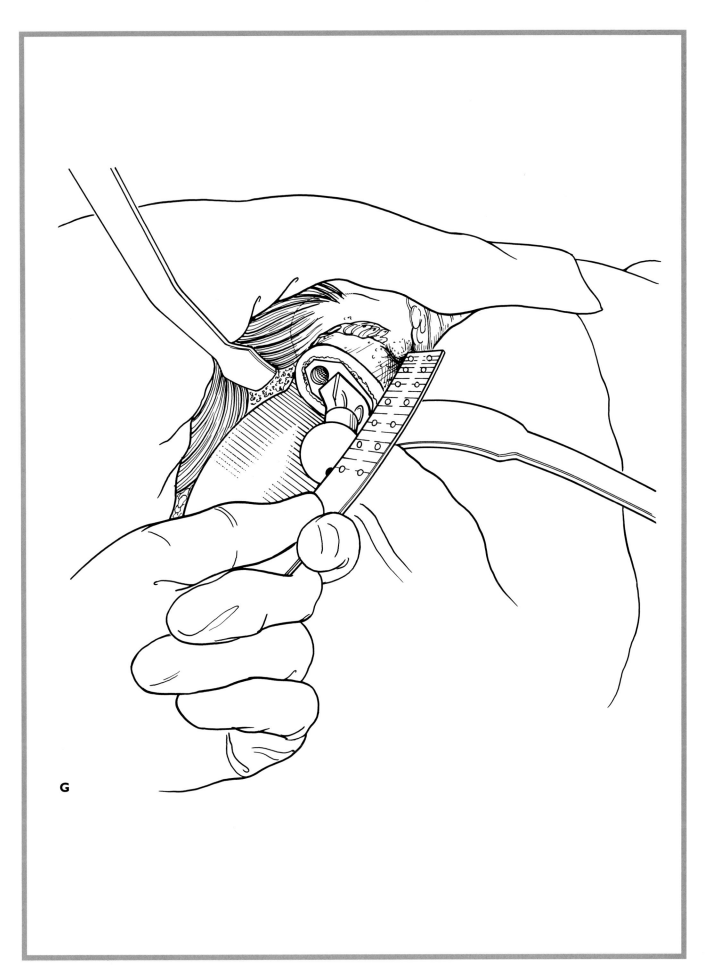

G

Trial Reduction

A.

A trial reduction is carried out.

B.

The range of motion should be stable through a functional arc. Posterior instability should be assessed with flexion, and internal rotation and anterior instability with extension, abduction, and external rotation.

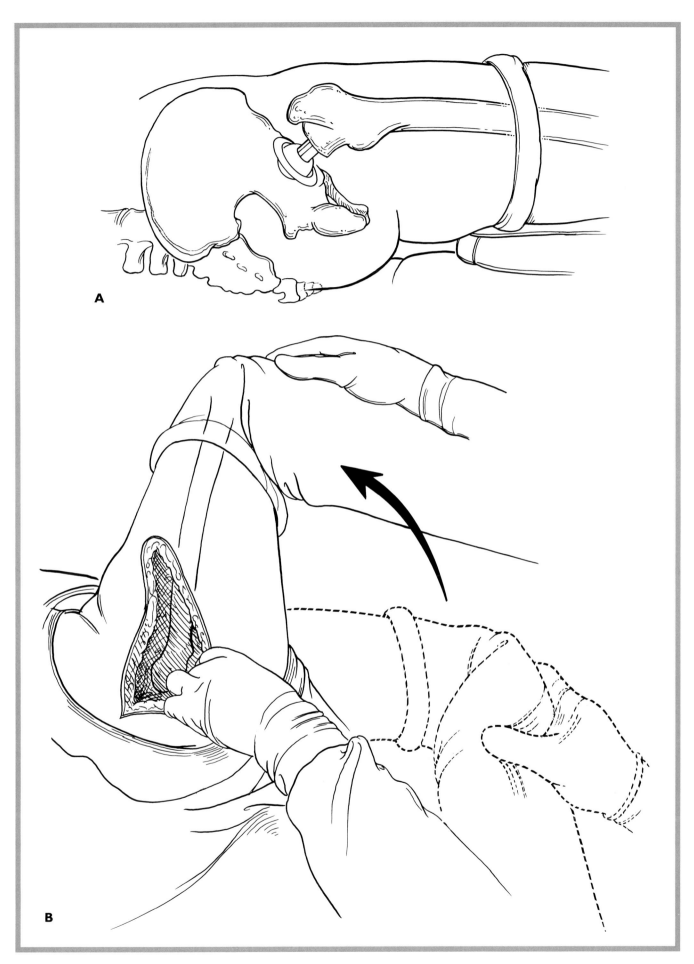

A

B

Broach Trial Removal and Femoral Component Preparation

A.

The hip is dislocated, and the broach trial is removed. In preparation for the final component insertion, the canal is suctioned and cleaned of any loose pieces of bone. It is important to remove all excess fluid and debris so that the component will seat properly.

B.

The distal tip is impacted onto the distal morse taper of the stem on the back table. The tip should be impacted forcibly. A polyethylene covered head impactor can be used.

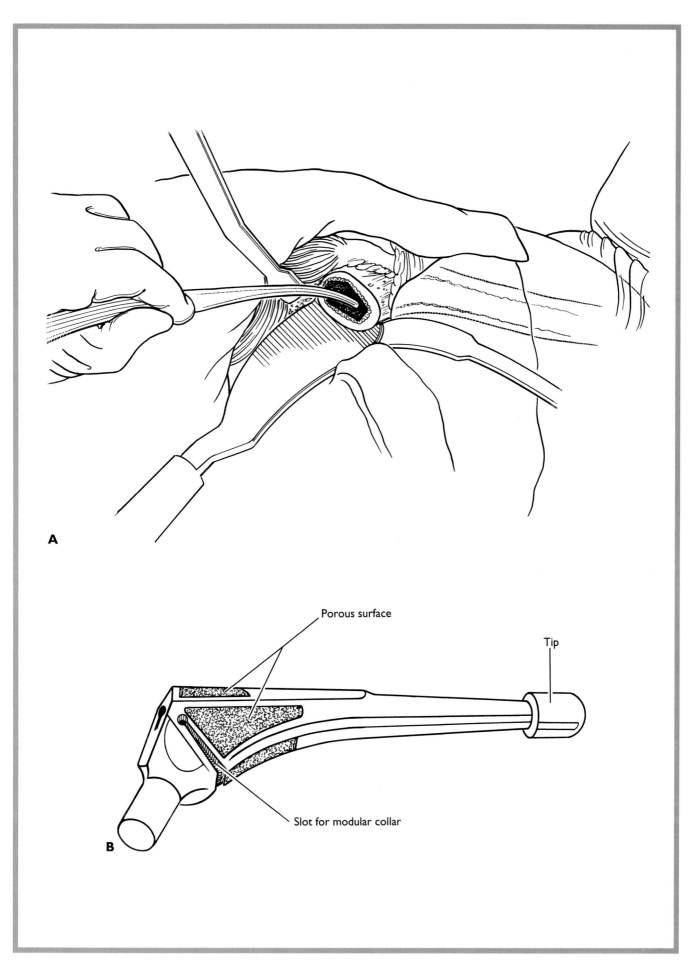

A

Porous surface

Tip

Slot for modular collar

B

12

Placement of Femoral Component

Femoral Component Placement

A.

The femoral component insertion handle is threaded into the femoral component.

B.

The component is impacted into the femoral canal. Resistance will be slightly greater than that encountered with the broach owing to the porous pads being slightly proud of the substrate surface. Owing to the viscoelastic properties of bone, component insertion over time should gradually improve. When using the distal tip on the stem, do not attempt extraction as this may lead to disengagement. The slot on the collar should approximate the cut of the femoral neck. If desired, one may use a modular collar in this implant.

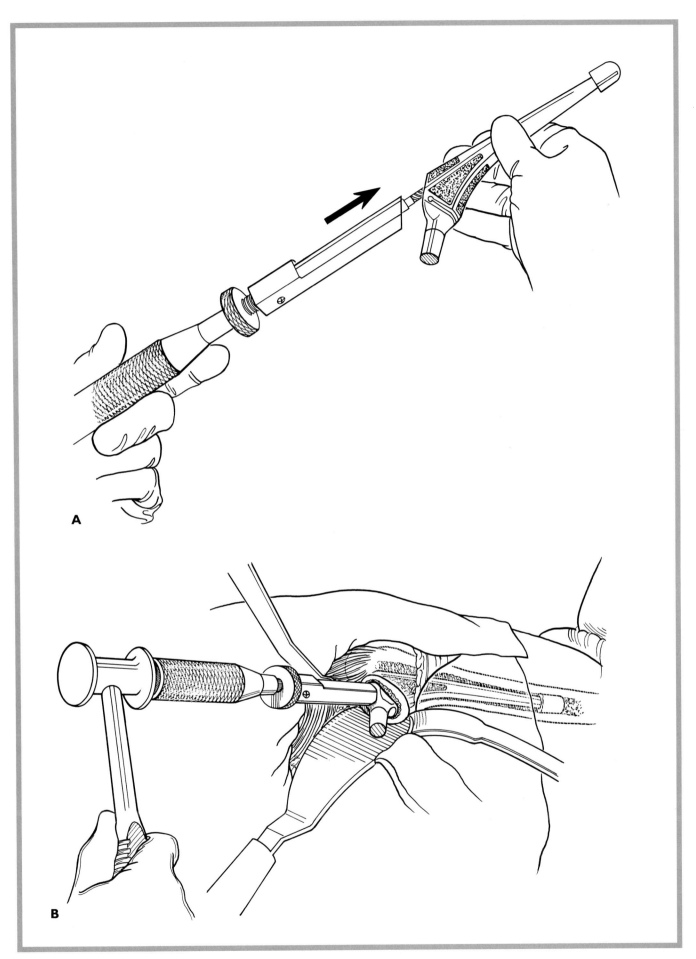

A

B

Trunion Preparation

The trunion is lavaged with sterile solution and dried. It is important that the trunion be clean and dry so that the head trunion couple is firm.

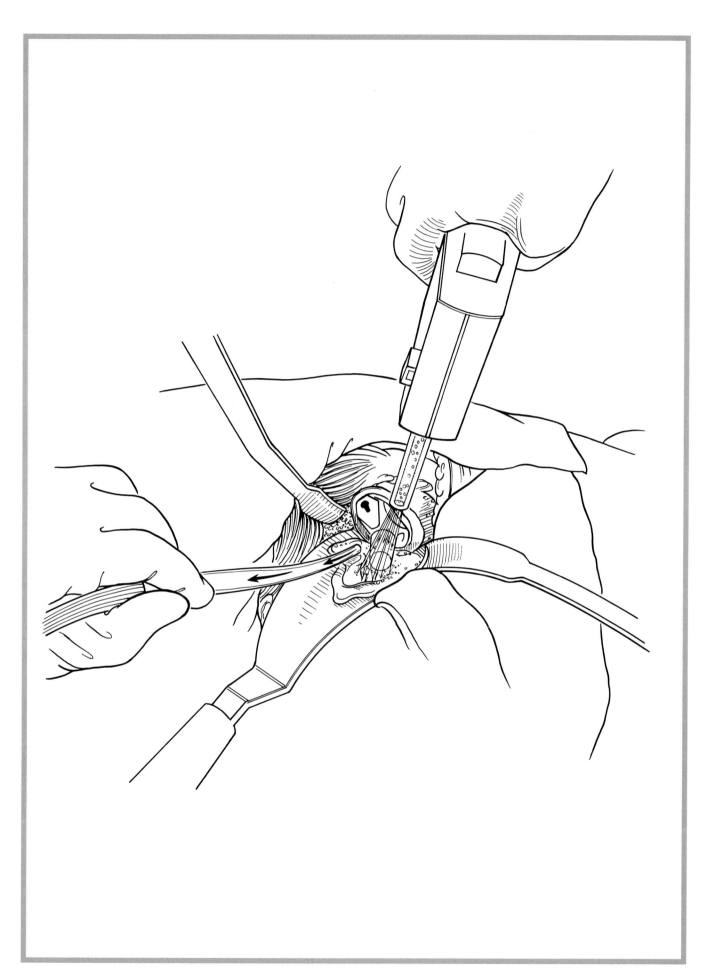

Head Impaction

A.

The head is gently impacted onto the trunion.

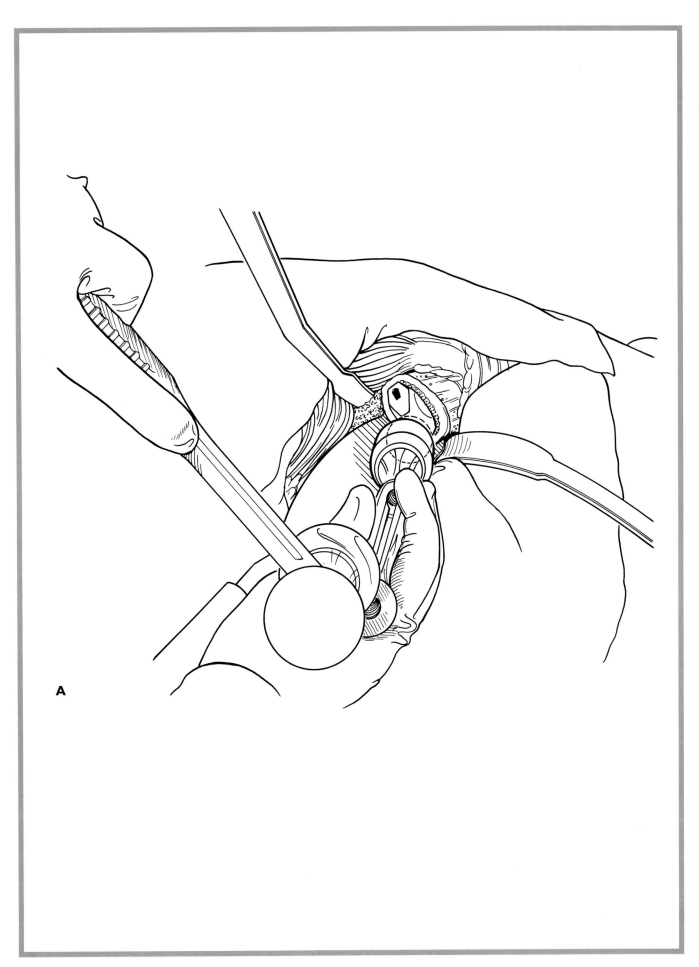

A

B.

An attempt is made to pull the head off to insure adequate fixation.

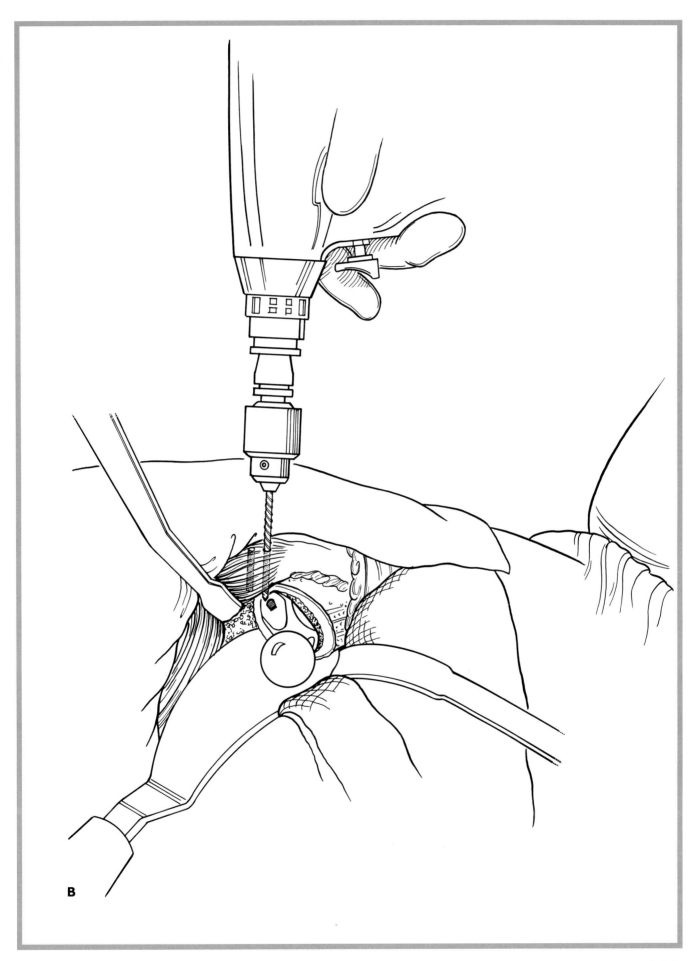

B

Index